D0306406

A Legal Framework for Caring

Also available from Macmillan:

Akinsanya, J., Cox, G., Crouch, C. and Fletcher, L. (1994) *The Roy Adaptation Model in Action*.

A Legal Framework
for Caring

An introduction to law and ethics in health care

Lucy Fletcher and Paul Buka

MACMILLAN

© Lucy Fletcher and Paul Buka 1999

All rights reserved. No reproduction, copy or transmission of this publication may be made without written permission.

No paragraph of this publication may be reproduced, copied or transmitted save with written permission or in accordance with the provisions of the Copyright, Designs and Patents Act 1988, or under the terms of any licence permitting limited copying issued by the Copyright Licensing Agency, 90 Tottenham Court Road, London W1P 9HE.

Any person who does any unauthorised act in relation to this publication may be liable to criminal prosecution and civil claims for damages.

The authors have asserted their right to be identified as the authors of this work in accordance with the Copyright, Designs and Patents Act 1988.

First published 1999 by
MACMILLAN PRESS LTD
Houndmills, Basingstoke, Hampshire RG21 6XS
and London
Companies and representatives
throughout the world

ISBN 0–333–72778–9

A catalogue record for this book is available
from the British Library.

This book is printed on paper suitable for recycling and
made from fully managed and sustained forest sources.

10 9   8   7   6   5   4   3   2   1
08 07 06 05 04 03 02 01 00 99

Editing and origination by
Aardvark Editorial, Mendham, Suffolk

Printed and bound in Great Britain by
Antony Rowe Ltd Chippenham, Wiltshire

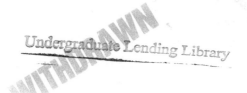
Undergraduate Lending Library
WITHDRAWN

For Brian and the Leonards
Carol, Sandy and Tinashe

Contents

Contents

Contents

Acknowledgements

The authors of this book wish to thank all those who have so patiently helped us. We have been lucky to have had the support of our colleagues and friends, particularly Andrea, Ruth and Julia, who listened to us when it was going well and helped us through the sticky patches. We wish to acknowledge the valuable guidance that we have received from Richenda Milton-Thompson.

A big thank you must go to the pre-registration students of all disciplines and to those studying for the NVQ who read drafts of the chapters, assessed them for their usefulness and also proof-read the work. Our thanks must also go to the librarians who helped us to find obscure works and recommended others that might be of use.

We owe a debt of gratitude to ARD, Karen Law, Phillip Ojianko, and Susan and Claire Soper for their expertise and assistance with various aspects of the book.

Preface

During the late 1980s and 90s, there were many changes in the legal framework of health care in the UK that have had an effect on the delivery of care. A radical reform of the National Health Service (NHS) has taken place over the past decade, allied to an increasing emphasis on care in the community by a multidisciplinary team working in collaboration for the benefit of its clients. A knowledge of the law and its basis is a vital part of the background and everyday practice of those who deliver health care to client groups.

Every effort has been made to ensure that the law quoted at the date of writing is correct. It is important to emphasise that this book is not intended to take the place of qualified legal advice or of that of trade union officials representing their members within the workplace. This book is designed to raise awareness of the relevant legislation and act as an introduction to the huge range of excellent texts that are available at a more advanced level. Each chapter is concluded by a section devoted to references and further reading relevant to the material contained within the chapter.

To simplify the learning process, case law has not been discussed as each case is judged on its individual merits and only a few keynote court decisions have been mentioned in the text. These decisions have come to form part of the everyday reference to the law made by health care professionals, and a fuller understanding of the process by which they have been determined will repay the more advanced student. Some of the care situations outlined are evolving within the law, the subject of euthanasia and the making of an advance directive (living will) being examples, so can only be discussed within the context of the law at the time of writing. Four chapters are devoted to general issues, with five discussing the law in relation to specific client groups. Addressing specific client groups has led to some duplication, for example in consent to treatment and duty of care, but this has been done in order to allow each chapter to stand alone within its client group.

The increasing use of technology in the workplace and an acknowledgement of the need for good record-keeping has resulted in further legal implications for those who deliver care. The rights of patients and their carers have now been identified, and the recognition by clients and their relatives of their rights with regard to health care have raised expectations of the expected standard of care. The right to complain about care and an increasing tendency to go to litigation are features of contemporary health care delivery to which the health care worker's only answer rests in the maintenance of full, accurate records.

Caring is closely linked to the related areas of morals and ethics, many of which affect both client and carer. This book concentrates on 'practical ethics', requiring the reader to link practice situations, that is, practical ethics, with the law within a caring situation. This takes the form of thinking points within each chapter related to the area under discussion, designed to stimulate thought and facilitate the transfer of theory to clinical practice. This approach is linked to the problem- and inquiry-based learning styles adopted within many educational courses at the present time. The thinking points have been extensively discussed by our students and colleagues in order to test their relevance, and their input was very valuable in the development of the book.

In order to ensure professional standards of practice and care, registered members of the multiprofessional caring team work within rules and codes of conduct developed by their professional bodies. The rules and codes form the yardstick for professional behaviour and standards both in the courts and for the professional bodies, and are briefly visited.

Changes, particularly in medical practice, have altered traditional patterns of accountability and responsibility, with consequent effects for all staff working with clients. The development of multidisciplinary care has resulted in a blurring of many of the former professional boundaries.

The importance of good communication and record-keeping is vital to permit effective co-ordination of the team members' work.

In this book, the terms 'health care worker' and 'health care professional' are used. 'Health care worker' relates to all those employed as paid carers, while 'health care professional' is used particularly in the context of the registered professional. The term 'client' has also been used unless the care setting is specifically within a hospital; this is to reflect the increasing emphasis on the care of all groups within the community.

Preface

Lucy Fletcher is a senior lecturer in nursing with a particular interest in the legal and ethical issues of care delivery.

Paul Buka is an experienced nurse and ward manager. He has a law degree and is currently undertaking legal studies at Master's level.

Chapter 1   Law and morals in society – an overview

Introduction

In most societies, the majority of rules, including legal ones, affecting citizens' lives have grown out of custom and usage, and are part of their heritage. Legal rules normally go through an assimilation process, having been influenced by whatever socio-economic, moral and other factors indirectly shape a particular society's ethics or rules of human behaviour. This includes its cultural and religious beliefs as well as those of its neighbouring societies, who may also influence it through social and political interaction. Given that man is not merely a thinking being, to counter the argument of some philosophers such as Descartes (1596–1650), human beings can be shown to be also moral beings. They are capable of discerning right from wrong, arguably according to the way in which they were bought up. There are no general moral standards of behaviour that are acceptable to all internationally: they vary from society to society since there is indeed no such thing as universal morality. In the UK, there is a basic presumption that all persons are equal before the eyes of the law and that the primary aim of the law is to protect its citizens and promote fairness. It is fair to say there are areas of consensus in which most societies accept that an action, for example one person intentionally killing another, is wrong. However, morality and the law are concerned with what a specific society views as right or wrong. 'Morality is concerned with right and wrong, good and bad, virtue and vice; with judging what we do and the consequences of what we do' (Nuttall 1995, p. 1); in the broadest sense, ethics is the outcome of a combination of the rules laid down by law and the associated morality of the society in which we live. The place of morals in society is to set acceptable standards of behaviour. The purpose of the law is to ensure fairness so that the weaker members of society are not compromised. In presenting evidence in any given case, the court must at times look to morals for guidance, as they are the fabric of our society. The court may question whether a defendant/defender's behaviour in a given situation matched that of the 'reasonable' man. The law is there not to apply purely the standards of the lawyers, but to look at the morals of the society where it developed.

When carers are faced with ethical choices or problems that cannot be resolved immediately, they may look to the law; similarly, registered professionals may consult their code of professional conduct, or local policies and guidelines, for the behaviour expected of them. In some situations, however, it is possible that they may face dilemmas that they cannot resolve, as discussed by Tschudin (1993, p. 134) In the UK, the traditional paternalistic view of care allowed the professional, in particular the doctor, not only to prescribe, but also to dictate care in the patient's interests. On the other hand, the spirit of the NHS and Community Care Act 1990 means that, to a large extent, patient autonomy should be the guiding factor when prescribing and providing care in the community, and discharge plans should be made accordingly. This means that clients have a right to lead an independent life at home and to determine their destiny within reasonable limits. In practice, the multidisciplinary team of professionals should work towards that goal in partnership with the client. The term 'professional' applies to both registered professionals and other paid carers who give care both in establishments and in the client's own home.

The moral argument that care should be provided at whatever cost is not realistic. In financial terms, the standard practice involving the internal market within the National Health Service (NHS) is that money should follow the patient. It is accepted that, when planning the delivery of care, the limited resources argument should be taken into account while working within the constraints of the law. The borders of morality and benevolence, doing good for the client and what the health care worker or carer could do for the client are boundless. In practice, the reality of the matter is that the moral argument cannot often win the day. From the point of view of the client, the question is how far the issue of morality should determine the kinds of law, and the quality of care and how it is delivered. NHS Trusts have to accept that resources are limited, and managers have to prioritise. There may be times when harsh decisions have to be taken as Trusts must live up to their financial responsibilities (that is, to deliver care within budget) and accountability. Financial management decisions sometimes conflict with ethical considerations when decisions are taken in rationing care. When that situation occurs, it is sometimes unrealistic for the law to be expected to intervene where resources are not limitless. Professionals should be guided by the supposition that, in a given situation, they will have acted in the patient's best interests given the constraints of available resources, and will have acted in accordance with legal requirements, professional rules and local policies.

However, moral values cannot be taken for granted (that is, they are not necessarily part of the law) when applying the law, as legal systems of different societies can often be seen to conflict, although morality seems to have a more universal appeal. This conflict has been the cause of religious strife and the basis of crusades both in the ancient and the modern senses. Most religions see it as their responsibility to teach morality. In Christian societies, of which the UK is one, laws have been substantially influenced by religion in areas such as family law, property law and the law of succession, in addition to canon (Church) law itself. One of the reasons for this influence is historical. Monks were among the few learned people who could read and write. The influence of the Church as property owners, administrators and owners of estates during the developmental feudal period was extensive. If one poses the question of what the essence of law is, there is no direct answer, only the fact that the law is seen as a system or body of rules that are prescribed by an authority of some kind in order to regulate human behaviour. It is also important that the effects of making laws are to have sanctions, or those laws will be ineffective. As to the question of what would happen to a group of individuals or a society that was not subject to any rules or laws, the answer is that there would be chaos, with survival of the fittest, who would thrive at the expense of the weakest members of that society. One could argue that this is a realistic situation. The difference that the law makes, however, is that it sees all people as equal. A useful definition of the law is 'Those rules which the courts will enforce' (McLeod 1996, p. 3). Once one has established what law is, the view that all persons are equal before the eyes of the law must be qualified by the reality that individuals have certain competing rights and obligations that the law can enforce.

Law and morality

Legal rules must be distinguished from what are society's moral values, which may be based on religion, custom or practice. There are nevertheless areas of common ground between the two. The laws of the UK have been influenced by the feudal system concerning the ownership of property as well as by the religious values that govern morality. Moral values should not be taken for granted to be hand in glove with the laws of any given country. For example, UK society may consider it immoral not to 'honour thy father and mother', yet, in fact, one cannot ask the courts to enforce this moral value as such, important though it may be to the fabric of society. The application of individual moral values depends on how a person's upbringing has instilled the ideas of the difference between right and wrong. Where religious values seem to be merged with morality, as in some religiously zealous countries, all law is seen as identical to, and deriving from, a divine source. History has seen that, at the other end of the spectrum, lie individuals with strong moral convictions who were following their consciences when they were prepared to die for their strong beliefs; here secular – man-made – law is subject to, and in conflict with, divine law. Examples are Thomas More (1478–1535) and John Fisher (1469–1535), who were martyred for upholding their moral beliefs that the king's laws could not supersede divine law and that they were subject to divine law in questioning the king's right to be the supreme head of the Church. The Abortion Act 1967 and the Human Fertility and Embryology Act 1993 are at present the only statutes that will make exceptions to the rule, for conscientious objectors.

In normal circumstances, moral values are imposed on the individual by family, Church, peer group or a professional body that attempts to control behaviour to curb excesses by developing a code of ethics – the product of moral belief. Any non-compliance is not normally enforceable by the courts unless it also involves a breach of the law.

The main difference between the law and morality is that while the former is enforceable in court, the latter does not necessarily attract legal sanctions. The rule, or authority, of law is symbolised by the visible machinery of the legal justice system – the arm of the law – comprising the police, the courts and the penal system. There are other aspects of the law to consider that affect not only our daily living – private and family law – but also our working lives. Jowell and Oliver (1994, p. 72) define the authority of the law as 'a principle of institutional morality. As such it guides all forms of law-making enforcement.'

The relationship between the object of the law and that of morality has been the subject of debate for centuries by scholars such as John Stuart Mill (1806–73) who saw the primary object of the law as being an ethical one, that is, to prevent harm to others. One theory of ethics, the utilitarian principle, could be used to describe the law as 'the greatest happiness for the greatest number of people' (Lee 1990, p. 22).

Our everyday lives are so embroiled in different aspects of the law that we cannot get away from its prescriptive nature as it sets standards of behaviour in order to encourage us to do good and ensure fairness. This democratic and populist view is supported by the stance of the positivist school of ethics that law is 'simply whatever is commanded by whoever happens to have the attention and obedience of most of the population' (Waldron 1990, p. 33).

The idea that there is a relationship between law and morality is supported by the natural law school, who put forward the proposition that no law is good law unless it conforms to the morality that we learn by our very nature. This then brings to the forefront the question of whether the caring relationship should be guided by purely ethical considerations. Where there is conflict between morality and law, for example on issues of abortion or euthanasia, health care professionals may find themselves at variance with the law. In situations such as this, the law sometimes makes allowances for conscientious objectors, as is given within the Abortion Act 1967.

The natural law school of thought considers that no law is good law unless it is in harmony with morality. This brings us to the issue of whether a caring relationship could be based on purely legal obligations and to what extent moral or ethical considerations should be allowed to influence it or to play a part. There is an inevitable overlap between morality and the law.

Thinking point

> Anne, a shop assistant in a small corner shop, is paid a meagre wage and finds it hard to make ends meet. She steals a loaf of bread to feed her family and is caught in the act.
>
> John is a well-paid accountant for an international company. He steals £2m over some years to finance an expensive lifestyle and has now been discovered.
>
> Is there a moral difference between the two? What is the similarity in law?

In general, the caring relationship is divided into formal and informal care. The first category usually comprises paid health care professionals who are supported by health care assistants, while the second category is composed mostly of unpaid relatives or friends who assist the dependent individual with personal or social care. In terms of professional carers, the law regulates how care should be delivered and affects systems of work when there are moral and ethical decisions to be made. This is particularly the case when one tries to establish a balance between the client's interest and the reality of limited resources while still preserving the moral considerations, which may shift and change at different times.

The basis of UK law

As seen above, the background of UK law has been shaped by both socioeconomic and historical factors. It can be seen in English property law that the interests of the landlord were safeguarded with regard to the rights of the landlord to repossess a property when the tenant was in breach of tenancy provisions. In the same vein, under Scottish law, more consideration is shown to the tenant.

The fusion of the regional legal systems as the UK became a national system was a result of the Acts of Union of 1536 and 1542 for England and Wales. The Act of Union of 1706 extended the union to Scotland, with Northern Ireland joining in 1800. In practice, Scotland, and to a lesser extent Northern Ireland, has in some respects retained independence within the legal system. Devolution for Scotland and Wales will change the balance of power as well as Westminster's law-making role. Under the plans, the Scottish parliament will have tax-raising powers and responsibility for all government business apart from defence, foreign policy and major constitutional matters. The Welsh Assembly, although having control of regional issues, is not to be empowered to raise taxes. The Channel Islands are subject to UK law in most respects, other countries that are colonies and protectorates, for example Montserrat in the West Indies and Gibraltar, also being subject to UK legislation.

Sources of Scottish Law

Scottish law has derived from a number of sources. The first of these is Roman law, going back as far as the Roman era. Second is canon (Church) law, which, although having influenced family law, succession law and property law, is itself effectively obsolete apart from within the Churches. Third, English law has influenced Scotland through business and academic exchange. The fourth source is institutional law, being unique to Scotland and based on the writings of respected scholars such as Professor Erskine, the Institutes (1773) and Viscount Stair's Institution (1681). Since the Union Act, Scottish law has developed with areas in common with English law, particularly in the areas of commercial law, as trading between Scotland and England was geographically inevitable.

To understand the basis of Scottish law, it is helpful to look briefly at the historical background of the Kingdom of Scotland that was established during the feudal period. Its beginning is usually associated with the battle of Cartham (1018), and it extends to the wars of independence between England and Scotland. During this time, Scottish law looked for the influence of other nations, in particular France, whose legal systems were influenced by Roman law. The feudal laws of both England and Scotland were, until the Reformation, largely a result of the influence of the Church.

Following the union of parliaments in 1707, the House of Lords became the final Court of Appeal for Scottish Civil Cases. The effect was that English law was applied to Scottish cases. In criminal law, appeals continue to be heard in the Scottish Court of Appeal.

Sources of UK law – the broader aspect

The laws of the UK as a whole derive primarily from two main sources. The primary source is parliamentary legislation from both the UK parliament and the European Community (EC).

The secondary source covers all other sources that have influenced and shaped the law and continue to give it its essence. This includes delegated legislation, that is, subordinate laws passed by bodies empowered by parliament to do so. Also included is the other class of 'quasi-legislation', which includes rules and regulations made by associations who are granted or delegated that authority by Royal Charter, but these are limited to certain groups and do not apply to all citizens. This is the class to which professional bodies belong, and under this provision, they may make rules that bind their members. In health care, these are the professional bodies such as the United Kingdom Central Council for Nursing, Midwifery and Health Visiting (UKCC) and the Royal College of Chartered Physiotherapists. Although their rules do not have the force of law in regulating general behaviour, they bind the practitioner through professional codes of conduct. These standards are adopted by the employer of the professional concerned. The professional codes are closely linked to morality – the rights and wrongs of professional behaviour – and are the expression, a code of ethics, of that right and wrong. The codes are also closely linked to the general law.

The European Community

Parliament, for the time being in respect of England and Wales together with Scotland and Northern Ireland, consists of the Queen as Sovereign, the House of Commons and the House of Lords. Since the UK became part of the then European Economic Community in 1973 on signature of the Treaty of Rome, we are now also bound by European laws and treaties. The European Communities Act 1972 incorporated EC law into that of the UK statute book.

There are four EC political institutions:

1. The *Council of Ministers*, which is made up of a group of ministers representing each of the individual member states. This is the most effective group insofar as it makes the EC laws
2. The *Commission*, which is to a degree the equivalent of the civil service and is responsible for making policies, which are subject to the approval of the Council of Ministers. It is there to support the Council of Ministers, although there have in the past been problems with Commission presidents not agreeing with the Council.
3. The *Assembly* – sometimes known as parliament – which is not a law-making body as its remit is mainly advisory to the Commission and it is run on the basis of consensus politics.
4. The *European Court of Justice*, not to be confused with the European Court of Human Rights, which is the highest court in the EC. It is responsible for interpreting EC laws and hearing appeals from member states. The judges, who are representative of the member states, are appointed for 6 years.

Article 189/EC defines the method, extent and application of European laws. The effect of EC membership is that, in the event of conflict between EC legislation and UK legislation, the former must prevail (Hill 1994, p. 6). EC law is applied in the European Court of Justice and appeals lie in that court, although it does not include constitutional law issues (Alder 1994, pp. 90–1).

There are three classes of European law: Regulations, Directives and Decisions.

1. *Regulations* must be applied directly in their entirety; that is, they have a general application to all member states.

2. *Directives* must be applied to bring national law into line with a timetable for implementation. An example of this is the Consumer Protection Act 1985, which protects the interests of the consumer against those of the seller and includes hire purchase and credit regulation.
3. *Decisions* are decisions of the European Court on appeal, which must be followed by the UK and the courts of member countries in respect of the parties or individuals to whom they are addressed. The validity of UK laws is based on the constitutional principle of 'parliamentary supremacy', that is, that parliament can make or unmake any laws it wants. This is now modified by EC membership.

Classification of law

The law is usually divided into the following classifications:

- *Public law*, which includes public international law. This deals with relationships between the state and its citizens, as well as interstate relationships. Examples are criminal law and constitutional law.
- *Private law* (civil law), which deals with obligations between private citizens. This includes employment law, tort and, in Scotland, delict and contract law, as well as family law. Private law is the main area of law that affects the caring relationship.
- *Substantive law*, dealing with the rules and procedures of law, which is a discipline based on historical principles and statutes. Examples are criminal procedure and civil procedure law. The main difference between criminal and civil law is that a crime is a wrong against the Queen's peace being punishable by sanctions imposed by the state. A civil wrong is one against an individual citizen and has to be pursued by the aggrieved individual in the courts.
- *Common law*. The law common to England and Wales has developed as its core a configuration of Norman law and local customs that were influenced by three sources: Danelaw, which prevailed after the Danish and Scandinavian invasions of the country; Mercian law, Germanic in origin and following colonisation by the Saxons; and Wessex law, derived from regional law in southern and western England.

In practice, English common law has also been influenced by the courts. This is an important secondary source of law that is the domain of the courts, as judges 'make' law. This is the area of 'judge-made' or case law in that the judge interprets and applies it to each individual case. In time throughout the development of the UK, the courts have had this role and continue to interpret and apply the law. The decisions of eminent judges have come to be followed as authoritative precedents, which means that they are binding to the lower courts and are treated with respect by courts of equal jurisdiction.

The other type of judge-made law in both English and Scottish law is called 'equity'; this has developed as 'residual' justice filling in the gaps where the strict application of legal rules could result in injustice for the individual seeking redress. The courts can use their discretion in applying this alternative 'equitable' principle. Equity as the king allowed his subjects to come forward with cases in which the litigants felt that they had been unfairly treated, to appeal to the King's conscience for 'residual justice'. In this situation, the normal rules of procedure did not apply, and justice was dispensed on the basis of fairness. In time, the king dedicated this role to an officer of the law, who became known as the Lord Chancellor, the 'King's conscience', who dispensed natural justice. Equitable principles were developed and relied on, and are now applied in the same civil courts by judges.

The justice system

The modern courts of the UK are divided mainly into the criminal and civil jurisdiction. The court system of Wales has been an integral part of the English system, while the Treaty of Northampton in 1328 conceded the independence of Scottish courts. For the purposes of this work, reference will be made mainly to civil law, although it is possible for an individual in breach of criminal law, for example one found guilty of rape, also to be sued for civil damages.

Magistrates Courts are the most important courts, dating back to the 13th century, when justices were appointed by the king (now by the Lord Chancellor's department) to keep the king's peace, hence the title 'Justice of the Peace'. The Magistrates Court has both civil and criminal jurisdiction. Civil jurisdiction relates to family law proceedings and local government matters, for example licensing law. There are both legally qualified 'stipendiary' magistrates and 'lay' magistrates sitting in the Magistrates Court. The lay magistrates should be seen as peers by those seeking justice. The Magistrates Court hears cases of first instance, which account for up to 95 per cent of all court cases. There is an appeal panel for this court, although there are few appeals. Magistrates also hear commital proceedings, which are preliminary proceedings prior to an expected commitment to a Crown Court. The distinction between the courts becomes more definitive as they reach a higher level.

Criminal jurisdiction

Criminal cases are normally initiated by the state, which means that the police, through the Crown Prosecution Service or the Procurator Fiscal in Scotland, take up the case on behalf of the Crown or the state. The burden of proof lies with the prosecution, who must prove their case beyond reasonable doubt, leaving no doubt in the mind of the judge or jury.

The Crown Court/Sheriff Court (Scotland) is normally the next court where appeals from the Magistrates Court can lay, as well as being the court of first instance dealing with more serious crime, for example armed robbery but not including murder and rape. Trial is by jury, with a panel of 12 jurors in England and Wales, and 15 in Scotland. The jury is drawn from the public at large via the Register of Electors for each district. In Scotland, the Sheriff Court has a wide jurisdiction in both civil and criminal matters. Appeals can only be against conviction, sentence or both but not against acquittal. Magistrates may also sit on the appellate bench in the Crown Court on appeal cases from the Magistrates Court. The High Court is responsible for trying the most serious crimes, such as murder and rape.

The Court of Appeal (criminal division) is where appeals from the Crown Court are normally heard by three judges in the presence of legal counsel only. Appeals against Court of Appeal decisions may be given leave to approach the House of Lords for a judgement.

In Scotland, appeals from the Sheriff Court lie in the High Court of Justiciary, in which the whole bench of judges may sit, and do not go to the House of Lords as in England and Wales. It is also important to note that, while in England and Wales, a defendant may be found guilty or not guilty of the charge, in Scotland there is also a 'not proven' verdict if the prosecution fails to establish their case.

Civil jurisdiction

In civil jurisdiction, the action must be brought by a citizen to claim for a remedy, usually money paid as damages, against another party. The burden of proof is much lower and must be proved on a balance of probabilities.

The Magistrates Court has civil jurisdiction as the court of first instance in family and licensing law. The County Court is also a court of first instance and, in addition, acts as a limited Appeal Court in some civil matters. Examples of County Court cases are actions for debt in the Small Claims Court.

The High Court/Court of Session (Scotland) deals with unlimited claims for damages under the law of contract as well as tort (or delict in Scotland), dealing with negligence. It also deals with appeals and administrative issues, and procedural matters such as injunctions, which are court orders preventing a named person from taking certain actions. In Scotland, the Court of Session can exercise its *'nobile officium'*, that is, its special function in the application of equitable principles. The Court of Session is the supreme civil court, being divided into the Outer House and the Inner House; they may also give permission for appeals to be heard in the House of Lords.

Certain appeals from the House of Lords can then, with leave of the House, be referred to the European Court.

Legislation and formal rules governing the caring relationship

A whole range of laws and regulations, as well as aspects of tort law (delict in Scotland), affect the caring relationship within both the formal, that is, paid, and informal, unpaid sectors of care.

In the formal care sector within the health care services, much of the existing framework of care is determined by existing government policy and statutes such as the NHS and Community Care Act 1990 and Department of Health (DoH) guidelines, which are updated regularly. Employment arrangements fall under employment law in general and are applicable to health care workers in both the public and private sectors of employment. In both public and private sectors, the professionals' and health care workers' conduct is governed by a contract of employment, a professional code of conduct, and, overall, by statute. One example is the Nurses, Midwives and Health Visitors Act 1972 as amended by the 1992 Act, whose main aim is 'To establish and improve standards of training and professional conduct for nurses, midwives and health visitors' and from which the current *Code of Professional Conduct* derives. The nurse will also have a contract of employment, under which both parties must satisfy their contractual obligations, including responsibilities under the Health and Safety Act at Work etc. Act 1974. Employees are expected to work up to the terms and conditions set up in their contract of employment (Young 1992, p. 4). Many employers will, in addition to the contract, develop policies and guidelines that should facilitate the employees' compliance with those terms as well as enhance care and provide standards that can be audited if required.

The informal care sector, on the other hand, forms a large element of care in the client's home. This is difficult to account for as a spouse or children may take over the role automatically. Because of the informal nature of the caring relationship, there is unlikely to be any form of contract of employment. The difficulty in regulating this area is obvious.

Duty of care and clinical negligence

In English law, the term 'tort' is derived from the Latin *torquere*, meaning twisted or contorted. Tort is a civil wrong for which the court may award damages, in contrast to criminal offences, which are against the state and may result in imprisonment. From the point of view of Scottish law, delict is seen as the law of reparation that is responsible for making good whatever harm has been suffered by the victim of the wrong.

The law relating to negligence is based on tort/delict law, whose primary aim is to compensate the victim of the act. Keenan (1995, p. 410) states that 'The tort of negligence has three ingredients and to succeed in an action the plaintiff must show (i) the existence of a duty to take care which was owed to him by the defendant (ii) breach of such duty by the defendant and (iii) resulting damage to the plaintiff.' It should be noted that, in Scotland, the terms 'pursuer' (injured party) and 'defender' (alleged wrongdoer) respectively are used.

Additionally, employed carers may also find that, if they are in breach of their contract of employment, they can be sued for damages if the loss is a result of their negligent act or omission. Although the term 'medical negligence' is used with reference to negligent acts committed by a doctor or a member of the allied professions, it may be less misleading to use the term 'clinical negligence' when dealing with professional carers who may be in breach of the duty of care.

At law, clinical negligence is the same as any professional negligence that is based on a position of trust relationship. Because of the trust vested in the professional by the client, such as is obvious when dealing with the issue of confidentiality, the law expects more from the professional. The professional must always act in the client's best interest. In practice, however, difficulty may be experienced in ascertaining what the patient's best interests are, and it may be relevant in such a case to seek a judicial review. This is where the court will declare what action ought to be pursued. The courts are reluctant to intervene in such cases and will often only do so in cases involving life and death.

When an injured party considers suing for damages for any harm suffered, the burden of proof, according to law, lies with them. It must be said that burden of proof is easier in a civil court as it depends on a balance of probabilities (50 per cent versus 50 per cent), compared with a criminal court, where the case must be proved beyond reasonable doubt (100 per cent certainty) in order to secure a conviction. If the prosecution has not proved its case beyond reasonable doubt in criminal proceedings, the accused must be acquitted.

In a civil court, the victim must go through the process of proving to the court that there was a breach, that there was a causal nexus or link, and that they suffered as a result of the negligent act of the defendant. The process that the court requires is (Brazier 1995, p. 240):

1. Proof by the plaintiff (the victim who is suing) that he or she was owed a duty of care by the defendant and that the injury or loss was within the foreseeability of the defendant (that he or she would have foreseen the likelihood of harm); that is, there is predictability that someone would be injured as a result of the negligent action or omission.
2. Proof that there was a breach of duty on the part of the defendant and that, as a result of that breach, someone (in this case the victim) suffered harm or loss.
3. That there must be a causal nexus or connection between the act or omission and the harm or loss suffered, which must not be too remote.

The courts will also consider whether the damage is close enough, the issue of proximity and policy issues – that is, whether it is in the public interest to award damages, sometimes called the remoteness of damages.

Breach of duty of care can also result from a failure of defendants to carry out an action that they should have carried out. English law looks for *culpa* or blame, while Scottish law, on the other hand, puts more emphasis on reparation or compensation for the harm suffered. The general principle looks at restoring (by compensation) the injured party to the position he or she was in before the harm took place.

If ethical principles are applied to clinical negligence, failure by a professional to reach required standards that result in a breach of duty of care should be seen as a moral wrong. This could result in the moral ostracism of the offender but, as such, can only be sanctioned in court if the above criteria is satisfied. In addition to court action, the professional body to which the individual practitioner belongs may institute its own proceedings, which may result in professional disciplinary action. Furthermore, the employer may also sue the employee who is in breach of duty of care for civil damages as well as following disciplinary procedures under employment law.

Professionals will be judged by the courts according to the standards of their profession. This is called the Bolam test, following a case in which an anaesthetist successfully defended a malpractice action after it was established that he had followed established practice (*Bolam* v. *Friern Hospital Management Committee*, 1957, 1 WLR 582; 1957 2 All ER 118). It is easy to see the relevance of professional codes of conduct, as the courts are likely to examine the practitioner's conduct to see whether a reasonable professional member of that group would have acted in that manner.

Litigation, remedies and dispute resolution

Owing to the complexity of this area, it can only be examined in outline. It is clear that, under the present UK 'fault' system, victims of clinical negligence have an uphill struggle to prove their case, this then being followed by a lottery as to whether they will win any compensation. Many complainants are put off by costs and the length of time that it would take to sue. The introduction of a 'no win – no fee' system is seen as a chance to open up the system to all claimants regardless of their wealth. This system means that the lawyers get paid out of any award made to their client, usually on a percentage basis (at present 30–40 per cent) should they win their case. This means that individuals with a meritorious case do not have to worry about the costs providing the lawyers are prepared to take on their case, but those on the borderline, or with a complex case, could find it difficult to retain a legal representative.

There are also other less formal, out-of-court, means of compensation, but they tend to award relatively small amounts compared with court awards for damages. The court is also likely to take into account any of these payments when awarding damages.

- *Social security payments*, to which both employer and employee contribute, may be paid after a period of time when the employee is unable to work. Social security payments are also available for victims of violent crime.
- *Indemnity insurance schemes* may pay out agreed amounts for any liability incurred by the accused employer or professional. The insured person will have made payments under a contract. Many health care professionals, notably doctors and others in independent practice make contributions to an insurance scheme of this type, the major company involved being the Medical Defence Union.
- *Occupational pension schemes*. Some occupational pension schemes will pay out, if an injury or accident affects an employee within the scheme. If the disability is long term, a pension may be payable.

The Franks Committee (1957, Cmnd 283) recommended that there should be other means of resolving disputes apart from recourse to the courts. This has been implemented in public administrative law and land law tribunals, administrative tribunals also giving the unhappy claimant the chance to appeal within the system at a cheaper and faster rate. The Small Claims scheme, started in 1975, now allows for claims of up to £3000 to go to automatic arbitration. More recently, the Wolfe Report (Lord Chancellor's Department 1996, p. 183) recognised that there were problems caused by delays and proposed a fast-track system for lower claims in civil cases. Victims of clinical negligence can now claim for damages for personal injury of up to £15000 in the County Court. This effectively reduces costs and waiting time, as a case going to the High Court could take anything from 7 to 10 years.

Since 1995, the DoH has introduced pilot mediation schemes for medical negligence claims in East Anglia and Oxford, and more health authorities are using these. The Wilson Report (Department of Health, NHSE 1995) encouraged health authorities to use such systems for complainants in order to reduce litigation. It would be at such hearings that out-of-court settlements were likely to be concluded. The process of alternative dispute resolution usually involves a panel of independent professionals examining the merits of a case informally and then recommending a course of action in order to resolve the dispute. Their decision would not be binding at law, and the dissatisfied client could still pursue legal action. Under some legal systems, victims are entitled to unlimited access to their medical records, UK law allowing the process under the Access to Medical Records Act 1984.

Thinking point

> Jason, a junior doctor in Accident and Emergency, negligently makes a wrong diagnosis and gives an incorrect injection to Mr Jones, an 80-year-old man who has been the victim of a road accident.
>
> Mr Jones sustains permanent brain damage as a result and is now unable to look after himself.
>
> Consider the ethical and legal issues involved.

Informed consent and information

The client's perceived rights include that to informed consent, which is the subject of clients' complaints with regards to information about their treatment. Common law in tort clearly states that the professional has a right to withhold some or all of this information if it is in the patient's best interests to do so. The client does not have unlimited rights, and this right is not enforceable at law. The government has recently acknowledged that although patients have rights under the Patient's Charter, they also have responsibilities. The general legal assumption is that the law requires the client who is under care to be owed a duty of care by the carer. Under the rights created by law, the client can sue for damages when a breach of that duty has occurred. The professional's defence would be that he or she cared for the client according to standards acceptable to the profession – the Bolam principle – even if others might hold a contrary opinion.

A consensus of ethical issues

Ethical values are based on consensus and religious morals, influencing thinking and practice. Although these principles do not have the force of law, they are guiding principles that are treated with respect when ethical decision-making is required. There are four principles: autonomy, beneficence, non-maleficence and justice.

The principle of *autonomy* is one given particular prominence in modern health care. Autonomy is the principle by which a client is given sufficient information about health care and then permitted to decide for him- or herself about treatment. This principle is visited several times throughout the book, particularly in relation to informed consent. Adults without mental health problems should be able to understand the benefits and drawbacks of their planned treatment and care. Understanding will, however, involve a number of factors, for example educational level, will they fully understand the explanation? In one of the authors' experience, a female patient stated that her second hysterectomy had been much more successful than the first, raising the point that she had a poor understanding of both her own anatomy and the pre-operative instruction that she had received.

The principle of *beneficence* is concerned with the provision of benefit or beneficial treatment to a client, while, broadly speaking opposite to this, *non-maleficence* seeks to prevent harm to that individual. Important aspects of these two principles are that clients have both biological and psychological needs, and that harm could be caused to one or other of these. It is now well established that clients who require surgical treatment recover better and experience less pain if both their physical and psychological needs are met. Thus the two principles can be seen to work together, physical and psychological preparation together with the surgery itself creating benefit, while the principle of non-maleficence is used in order to prevent complications.

The principle of *justice* within a health care context is more concerned with wider issues than those posed by individual clients and relates to broader matters. The ethical issues of resource allocation are often used to draw examples, which may concern either small or large groups. Media attention and social policy have been focused on the number of people on waiting lists for hospital treatment, and resources are periodically allocated by central government to ease the problem. Such funds must be found from somewhere. Is it better to withdraw funds from defence money in order to ease the waiting lists for health care? Initially, it would seem so, but what of the number of people and their families who are employed within the defence industry and who may lose their livelihood as a consequence?

Conclusion

The complexity of modern health care, and a public increasingly aware of its rights, requires all professional carers to have a knowledge of the law and the closely linked concepts of morals and ethics. As already discussed, 'morality is concerned with right or wrong, good and bad, virtue and vice; with judging what we do and the consequences of what we do. Moral philosophy, or ethics is that branch of philosophy which has morality as its subject' (Nuttall 1993, p. 1). While the law of the land applies to all citizens, and most people will have a fair idea of what is right or wrong – a sense of morality – codes of moral behaviour have been developed to guide professional practice. These codes of ethics, normally titled codes of conduct, allow the professional to judge what is right or wrong in professional behaviour towards clients and other professionals.

Health care professionals and workers are faced with moral dilemmas every day of their working lives, not perhaps the major issues used as a focus for examples but smaller and more individual matters. They will need to be fully aware of how existing rules expect them to work; they may have to resolve the question of how far a client should be pushed during rehabilitation or to what extent a client who refuses treatment should be pushed – if at all. Other questions arising could involve whether elderly clients should have drugs forced upon them – or disguised in jam; whether a child should be allowed to choose treatment; whether a mentally ill client should be allowed to lie in bed all day even if it will damage his or her health; and whether mentally handicapped clients should be taken shopping even if they are disruptive. It is decisions such as this that go to the core of practical ethics, described by Singer (1993, p. vii) as 'relevant if it is one that any thinking person must face', but which the law cannot necessarily resolve.

References and further reading

Alder J (1994) *Constitutional and Administrative Law*. Basingstoke, Macmillan

Beale A (1994) *Essential Constitutional Law*. London, Cavendish/CP Essential Law Series

Brazier M (1995) *Street on Torts*. London, Butterworth

Department of Health NHS Executive (1995) *Acting on Complaints: the Government Proposals in Response to 'Being Heard'* (The Wilson Report). London, HMSO

Dyer C (1993) *Doctors, Patients and the Law*. Oxford, Blackwell

Elliott C and Quinn F (1996) *Tort Law*. London, Longman

Hill B (1994) *The European Union* (2nd edn). London, Heinemann

Jowell J and Oliver O (1994) *The Changing Constitution*. Oxford, Clarendon Press

Keenan D (1995) *Smith and Keenan's English Law* (11th edn). London, Pitman

Lee S (1990) *Law and Morals*. Oxford, Oxford University Press

Lord Chancellor's Department (1996) *Lord Wolfe's Final Report to the Lord Chancellor on the Civil Justice System in England and Wales* (Wolfe Report). London, HMSO

McLeod I (1996) *Legal Method* (2nd edn). Basingstoke, Macmillan

Marsh S and Soulby J (1990) *Outlines of English Law* (5th edn). New York, McGraw-Hill

Marshall E (1995) *General Principles of Scots Law* (6th edn). Edinburgh, W Green/Sweet & Maxwell

Montgomery J (1997) *Health Care Law*. Oxford, Oxford University Press

Nuttall J (1993) *Moral Questions: An Introduction to Ethics*. Cambridge, Polity Press

O'Neill A and Coppel J (1994) *EC Law for UK Lawyers – the Domestic Impact of EC Law Within the UK*. London, Butterworth

Redmond P and Shears P (1993) *General Principles of English Law*. London, M & E Handbooks

Sheridan M and Cameron J (1992) *EC Legal Systems: An Introductory Guide*. London, Butterworth

Singer P (1993) *Practical Ethics* (2nd edn). Cambridge, Cambridge University Press

Tingle J and Cribb A (1995) *Nursing Law and Ethics*. Oxford, Blackwell Science

Tossell D and Webb R (1995) *Inside the Caring Services*. London, Hewer Text Composition

Tschudin V (1993) *Ethics in Nursing*. London, Butterworth Heinemann

Vincenzi C (1996) *Law of the European Community*. London, Pitman

Waldron J (1990) *The Law*. London, Routledge

Young A (1992) *Case Studies in Law and Nursing*. London, Chapman & Hall

Chapter 2 Caring within a framework

- Introduction
- The NHS
- Resources
- Employment and industrial relations
- The multidisciplinary team and codes of conduct
- Record-keeping
- Quality assurance in caring
- When it goes wrong – whistleblowing
- Complaints
- Research ethics
- Conclusion
- References and further reading

Introduction

The material in this chapter is principally that which affects the health care worker during his or her employment. The largest health care employer in the UK is undoubtedly the NHS, which at some time or other touches the lives of the vast majority of people living in this country. The development and current structure of the NHS are discussed, together with its legal basis and some resource issues affecting the organisation in the present climate. The effects of European legislation on the NHS are discussed briefly, but these are dealt with primarily in other chapters, particularly that which examines safety in care delivery (Chapter 4). Closely linked to the success or failure of any business, in modern parlance including the NHS, are the availability of resources and the costing of care, together with its effect on the individual, whether client or employee; consideration is therefore given to these issues. The reader will find that useful further reading is supplied by books on social policy and economics in addition to those from legal and ethical fields of study.

The majority of health care workers are employees either of the NHS or a private employer, and the place of industrial relations and practice is considered, together with the place held by the trade unions. Trade union membership is widespread within the NHS but arguably less so among the employees of smaller concerns. Trade unions do, however, play a significant part in the development of workplace practices throughout the country, many of which percolate from the larger employers to the smaller.

Professional bodies have a profound effect on the work of the individual practitioner and influence work practices in general. Although this influence is at its most intense for registered practitioners, those training for the professions must be fully aware of the demands of their professional codes or rules of conduct. As the codes and rules are produced by the registering bodies, infringement of the professional codes may result in deregistration of the practitioner, with consequent loss of status and earnings. The relationship of codes and rules of conduct to the law is considered, along with their significance for the expected professional behaviour of the practitioner.

Nurses may form the largest number of health care professionals in the delivery of care, but not all care is the province of nursing. Increasingly, the vital input made by other health care professionals, both in hospital and in the community, is a great part of the treatment and rehabilitation of the client. Thus as codes and rules of conduct are important, so is the smooth working of the multidisciplinary team in health care.

Quality assurance and the measurement of care-giving would seem difficult to quantify; much thought has been given to these over recent years, and systems have been developed in order to quantify the good and bad aspects of practice. Although these issues impinge more on the ethical than the legal side of care delivery, the widespread adoption of audit mechanisms and quality assurance methods makes their inclusion a topic of necessity.

Research is an essential feature of professional work and is now widespread within the health care professions. The place of research ethics and the ways in which clients' interests must be protected have been included as many health care workers, while not conducting research themselves, may know of colleagues who are working on a research project and should understand the ethical considerations that are part and parcel of research work.

Record-keeping, whether computerised or paper based, is, many would say, the bane of health care work. Despite this, record-keeping is extremely important and cannot be neglected; legal proceedings may take many years to come to court, memories fade, and all that may be left is the record made at the time of the incident. Records also allow for smooth handover either from one professional to another or to facilitate communication among different groups of professionals concerned with the care of one client. Records therefore form an integral part of care delivery.

Even in the best-regulated world, things can and do go wrong at times. Health care delivery is no exception to the rule, and all three parties involved – the employer, the employee and the client – may at some time have cause for complaint. As health care delivery presents a more and more commercial face, consumers are likely to feel an increasing freedom to complain about poor service, just as they would in any other commercial service provision. An increasing trend on the part of complainants to resort to litigation if complaints cannot be dealt with promptly and effectively makes effective complaints management a necessity.

The NHS

The NHS in the UK, with its ideology that health care for all should be free at the point of delivery, was 50 years old in 1998. Prior to the 1939–45 war, health care was arranged principally on payment for service unless the client could prove poverty or was a member of a workers' insurance scheme. Housewives, in an age where few married women worked, children, the elderly and the disabled received little health care; however, these are the very groups that, as social research has demonstrated, require the most help in health matters. During the interwar years, institutional health care was broadly divided into that delivered by the voluntary hospitals, supported by endowment or money raised by local people, and that provided by the municipal hospitals run by local authorities under the 1929 Local Government Act. In many areas of the country, this resulted in duplication, services being developed by both sectors to serve broadly the same population. This duplication of effort was to have long-lasting consequences, and was in some cases only settled during the hospital centralisation of the 1980s and 90s.

The inception of the NHS in 1948 was the result of the 1946 National Health Service Act. This Act is an example of how social enquiry and the resultant official reports may influence law. Changes in health care were first outlined in the 1942 Beveridge Report (see Webster 1988). A White Paper – a formal policy discussion document – entitled *A National Health Service* was issued in early 1944, setting out official government policy. Beveridge had recommended changes to the hospital service alone, but contributions and opinion from both interested parties and the public became incorporated into the White Paper. The result was a comprehensive health scheme involving both hospital and general practitioner services, with free treatment for all funded by taxation. The wartime coalition government then drafted the NHS Bill, which was considered by parliament initially in committee and then in the full House of Commons. In 1946, the Bill was passed in parliament, thus giving the date of the Act. As with any reforming legislation, time was needed after the passing of the Act in order for changes to be put in place, and a period of more than 2 years was given to allow for reorganisation. The 1946 NHS Act took effect in summer 1948 and began a new era radically different from the previous picture.

The later stages of the 1939–45 war saw the birth of much of the modern framework of both health and social care. During the immediate post-war period, the 1944 Education Act, the 1946 NHS Act, the 1946 National Insurance Act and the 1948 National Assistance Act were introduced. These Acts were designed to produce widespread social reform and to form the bedrock of the new post-war Britain.

Structurally, the NHS was designed to meet the needs of each of the four countries that make up the UK, each country's organisational base being rooted in appropriate legislation amended and updated as necessary. The organisational bodies are the National Health Executive (England), the Scottish Health Boards, the Welsh Health Authorities and, in Northern Ireland, the Health and Social Services Boards.

The NHS has taken action on reports that it commissioned in order to improve services or the use of resources; one example is the Griffiths report of 1988 (House of Commons Social Services Committee), which in due course laid the ground for the 1990 NHS and Community Care Act. Despite these and the introduction of the 'internal market' in the past decade, the fundamental philosophy of the NHS remains in that it should be free to all at the point of delivery.

In the same way as the original NHS Act of 1946, the current NHS legislation came into being over a period of years and in response to greater awareness of the benefits of care in the community for the sick and dependent. As with the Beveridge Report, the basic idea sprung from the Griffiths Report of 1988, commissioned by the Secretary of State for Health in 1986. The Report was followed by a White Paper *Caring for People: Community Care in the Next Decade and Beyond* (1989), and, after the parliamentary committee stages, was placed before the House of Commons, becoming the NHS and Community Care Act 1990, which came into force in April 1993. The Act sees a close link between hospitals, community health care workers and the social services in order to improve the provision of care, and places great importance on the assessment of a client's needs in the community. In the period between the passing of the Act in 1990 and its implementation in 1993, local authorities were required to develop community care plans to assess the level of requirement for their services within the population served.

The present government wishes to extend and further integrate health and social services to allow for more flexible care within the community. The plan for NHS reform within England was published in the White Paper *The New NHS: Modern, Dependable* (Department of Health 1997). This White Paper, together with the Primary Care Act 1998, and the eventual development of primary care Trusts by general practitioners, nurses and therapists working in the community, places emphasis on community-centred care as opposed to hospital-centred care for the future. Plans for Scotland are also identified in the White Paper *Designed to Care*, published by the Scottish Office (1997). The White Paper reviews the work of the Scottish Health Boards and, in a way similar to that of the English reforms, envisages the development of multidisciplinary primary care Trusts within Scotland.

Although not affecting the structure of the NHS, an important principle was addressed by the passing into statute of the National Health Service Amendment Act 1986. Passage of the Act removed the Crown Immunity previously enjoyed by hospitals in the UK. After the 1946 Act, the NHS, as a government body, had been considered to be an agent of the Crown and therefore immune from the enforcement of many areas of legislation. As the UK became increasingly subject to European law, and following on a number of publicised cases involving food safety in hospitals, Crown Immunity was removed by the 1986 Act. The Food Safety Act 1990 reiterates this in its classification of a business by including premises, for example hospitals, where food is supplied without charge, in this case to patients.

Resources

Although health economics are not the purpose of this book, some understanding of the ways in which both public – that is, NHS – care and private care are funded is useful for several reasons. The NHS is funded by taxation, giving all taxpayers an indirect interest in its general affairs. Financial matters have a knock-on effect on resource issues, for example staffing. Cases publicised in the media that involve ethical matters may have an underpinning resource argument, as has the development of health care 'rationing'.

The 1990 NHS and Community Care Act basically endorses the concept as it was originally envisaged – a service funded by the taxpayer. The concept brings forward one immediate economic difficulty in contemporary Britain, that of the rising age of the population. As more people live for longer in retirement, the tax product of their income is dropping and affecting the government's own income from taxation. Income from taxation is also affected by levels of unemployment. A falling taxation product not only affects the NHS, but also other taxation-based social welfare schemes such as the payment of old-age pensions and social security benefits. To meet this challenge, the NHS Executive, the Management Executive in Scotland and the Management Executive in Northern Ireland are constantly looking at ways in which the service can be made more efficient and costs saved in order to meet service demands.

As the source of NHS income remains taxation, the amount of funding awarded is subject to the will of the government in power following the budget debate in parliament. In each country, the allocated amount is made from the Executive to health authorities and Trusts. Each authority or Trust's allowance is calculated by reference to a formula including the numbers and ages of people served in order to meet its service requirement. The authority, in return, submits its planned spending target and is expected to meet budget targets.

Government plans published in the two White Papers – *The New NHS: Modern, Dependable* (Department of Health 1997) and *Designed to Care* (Scottish Office 1997) – are aimed at giving even greater responsibility to primary care providers, with doctors, nurses and therapists purchasing services to meet the needs of their client groups within the community.

The past decade has seen enormous strides made in health technology and treatment, and the consequent costs of delivering health care. Conditions can now be treated that were formerly intractable; aggressive treatments for diseases such as cancer and HIV have been developed to prolong life. Transplant surgery is becoming more commonplace. The use of electronic monitoring devices is a regular feature of care in both hospitals and the community. At the same time, the rising age of the population has demanded more care for the elderly in our society, placing a further drain on health care resources. These developments have resulted in increased costs to the provider of care and raise the ethical issue of health care rationing as resources become scarce. Decisions have to be made about who is to be treated and on what criteria candidates should be selected for treatment. Should age or expected outcome play a part in the decision-making? It is difficult decisions like these that have become part of health care in the current climate and in which health care workers may be involved.

Thinking point

Tim is 72. He has been a fit and active man, and often acts as a volunteer driver for the community bus. He and his wife care for their three grandchildren while their son and daughter-in-law are at work. Tim has suffered a myocardial infarction and subsequent cardiac arrest. Resuscitation was successful, and Tim now requires an urgent coronary artery bypass operation.

John is 36 and works full time; he and his wife have no children. He has a congenital condition that has resulted in his needing coronary artery bypass surgery, and it is now essential that he has the operation.

Which man should be operated on?

It is a situation such as the one outlined in this Thinking Point that illustrates the dilemma of modern health care. Both men are active and lead a full life. The main differential is their age, and this might be a factor in expected recovery and the success or failure of surgery. It is probable that the decision of whether or not to operate would be decided on an individual basis linked to the availability of skilled professional staff. Alternatively, the surgery could be carried out on a private basis if either man had the financial means to pay for it.

On the face of it, the private sector in health care is relatively straightforward. Money is paid in direct return for a service given, in this case health care. In most instances, the client is successfully treated and cared for, either returning home or continuing to reside in the home selected. However, for some, the money will run out, or they will develop further illness, and it may be the NHS or local authority that is left to provide for the client's needs. The changing transaction may bring with it an ethical dimension as the NHS is less and less able to meet the demands placed upon it.

Thinking point

> Ellie is 85 years old and has lived in a nursing home for 2 years. It is her stated wish that she should remain in the nursing home until she dies. She has recently become confused and has developed a chest infection. The on-call GP visits and wants Ellie to be transferred to the local hospital where she can be given oxygen and intravenous antibiotics. The doctor expects that she should subsequently recover from her illness.
>
> Ellie's relatives are aware of her wishes and oppose the transfer to the hospital. The nursing home staff are willing to continue to care for her but are unable to deliver the same level of intervention that would be possible in the hospital.

A scenario such as that in the Thinking Point above is not uncommon. Should Ellie be transferred to the hospital as the general practitioner feels that her chances of recovery are high? His wish is opposed by that of Ellie herself – who is now confused – and her family, who are aware of her previously stated wishes. The care at the local hospital is known to be good, and although the beds are under intense pressure, an immediate admission is poss-ible. The nursing home staff admit that they would be unable to deliver the same level of intervention that can be offered under the

NHS, although their basic care is of a high standard. In a situation such as this, what is decided may well become a matter of negotiation between those involved. On this occasion, Ellie's wishes were respected and she remained in the nursing home, but treatment was available within the NHS and could have been taken up.

Employment and industrial relations

The overwhelming majority of those working in health care are likely to work for an employer, independent professionals being in the minority. In such work, the terms 'employee' and 'health care worker/professional' have been used interchangeably to reflect the status of the majority in that they work for either an organisation – for example, the NHS – or a company as their employer. The employer pays wages or a salary and deducts tax and national insurance from the money paid. There will usually be a written contract of employment. Many health care workers are employed personally by an agency, while the agency itself is contracted to supply a service – its staff – to the business to whom it is contracted.

An individual independent contractor is contracted to provide a service. Contractors are usually paid in full for their services and must make their own arrangements for the payment of tax and national insurance. In health care, an example of this might be provided by a nursing home that contracts therapy services from a self-employed chartered physiotherapist in independent practice.

By the time someone applies for a particular job, the employer has usually devised a job description or job specification. The details normally specify the grade of staff required, management links and the place of work. In large organisations where pay is allotted to particular scales, the pay scale and pay rates are also included. An outline of the duties that employees will be expected to fulfil in the post for which they are applying is also a feature and allows candidates to assess for themselves whether or not they are able to meet the requirements of the post. The job description or specification is also of relevance if the employee is liable to dismissal on capability grounds by being unfit to do the job for which he or she was employed because of ill-health or injury. Although the job description does not form part of the contract of employment, it often forms part of the evidence used in industrial relations negotiations.

One of the key features of a contract is that there are two sides to the agreement, in this case the employer and the employee, both of whom have rights in law and both of whom are named in the contract. The contract of employment sets out the terms of service with the employer but may also determine the behaviour expected of employees in relation to the work they are to perform. In health care work, contractual behaviours are likely to relate to the maintenance of client confidentiality, together with clauses banning the employee from working while under the influence of either drink or drugs, and prohibiting theft from clients. The penalties for what is often termed 'gross professional misconduct' may include instant dismissal or suspension of employment until the behaviours are investigated and judged by a disciplinary hearing. For professionally qualified staff, behaviours such as those outlined above will almost certainly breach the professional codes of conduct, the professional then becoming liable for action to be taken not only by the employer, but also by the registering body.

In addition to expected behaviours, the contract of employment will specify the conditions of service under which the employee is to work in relation to hours to be worked, holiday entitlement, sick and holiday pay, and details of pension entitlement. Employers of more than 20 people will also have to specify in the contract what action is to be taken in the event of disciplinary proceedings or if a staff member has a grievance against the employer. Once appointed, or at least within 2 months of the commencement of employment, the employer must give the employee a written contract stating the terms of employment provided that the employee is to work for 8 hours or longer each week. 'This statement must contain the names of the employer and the employee; the date when the employment began; whether employment with a previous employer is to be counted as part of the employee's "continuous period of employment" and, where this is so, the date on which it began' (Keenan 1995, p. 319).

Conditions of service are controlled nationally by a number of statutes that govern employment law in the British Isles, ranging from the Employment Acts, the Sex Discrimination Acts of 1975 and 1986 and the Race Relations Act 1976. Employment protection is covered in the Employment Protection (Consolidation) Act 1978, and the activities of trade unions are governed by the Trade Union Reform and Employment Rights Act 1993. The Health and Safety at Work etc. Act 1974 and associated safety Regulations are also important components of employment, with rights and duties on the side of both the employer and employee. The employment of disabled people is covered by the Disability Discrimination Act 1995, and in this case the job description may be useful to both sides in outlining the duties that are to be undertaken by employees in the course of their work.

The Employment Protection (Consolidation) Act 1978, which governs employment rights in both England and Scotland, regulates the length of notice that an employer must give when terminating the employment, and this notice period should be included in the contract of employment. The Act also gives employees the right to appeal to an Industrial Tribunal if they feel that they have been unfairly treated and wish to apply for reinstatement.

The largest trade union in health care is UNISON, which represents many groups of health care worker, ranging from professionals of all types to unskilled staff. Specialist unions such as the Royal College of Nursing, the Royal College of Midwives and the Health Visitors Association represent their members as well as providing a professional support service.

Trade unions play a large part in collective bargaining, that is, representing the rights and interests of the mass of their members across the country to employers such as the NHS. However, as health care Trusts are likely to begin to develop their own employment and pay strategies, collective bargaining over conditions of employment is likely to change to a more localised pattern. On a local level, trade union activities and the representation of staff are undertaken by unpaid stewards, trained by the union, who will represent union members' interests in employment matters. A union steward will represent a union member's interest at disciplinary proceedings and when a genuine grievance against the conditions of work is made by the employee. Should the steward require help and advice, the union employs permanent officers to assist them on either a national or a regional basis. The work of union stewards is regulated by the Trade Union and Labour Relations (Consolidation) Act 1992. Under this Act, stewards are entitled to time off with pay both while they are undertaking their training and while carrying out official trade union work. The work of the steward can, for example, include representing either the entire membership or an individual member in negotiations with the employer.

Safety representatives are also trained by the unions to ensure that the workplace is safe to the standards of current legislation and that the health and safety at work requirements are met.

As there are two sides to the contract of employment, there may be reasons why one side or another wishes to end the contract. Should the employer be the party who ends the contract, notice must be given to the worker depending upon the length of service as ruled in the Employment Protection (Consolidation) Act 1978. In some cases, the employer may be allowed to dismiss the employee if the employer can prove that the dismissal is on the grounds of capability. When deciding capability, the employer must be able to show that dismissal is on the grounds of inability to do the job because of a lack of qualifications on the part of the employee and that further training has failed to improve performance. Other capability issues surround the dismissal of workers who are unable to do their job as a result of illness or injury if no suitable alternative employment can be found for them within the organisation. Fair dismissal by the employer may also be on the grounds of conduct, that is, unsuitable behaviour as outlined in the contract of employment, for example being drunk on duty or abusing clients. Genuine redundancy is also grounds for fair dismissal.

Employees who have been dismissed from their jobs may have grounds of appeal to an Industrial Tribunal, who will judge the case after hearing both sides of the argument. The Tribunal is composed of a legally qualified chairman who 'usually sits to decide the case along with two other persons; one person is drawn from employers' organisations and the other from trade union organisations' (McHale 1998, p. 4). At a Tribunal, the employee is normally represented by a solicitor who may be provided by a trade union if the employee is a member, or paid by the employee. At disciplinary hearings, the employee is represented either by the union steward or by another person who acts as a 'friend' but is not legally qualified.

Industrial relations is a very large branch of UK law, one in which the legal profession has members specialising in the work involved. Legal action is almost exclusively through the civil route and may therefore be expensive to the employee unless costs are awarded following what may be a protracted period.

The multidisciplinary team and codes of conduct

Modern health care has become increasingly complex and demanding in order to support clients, allowing them to achieve their maximum potential. Contributing to care are a number of different professional groups supported by students and workers studying for National Vocational Qualifications (NVQs), together with unqualified workers. The importance of what is known as the multidisciplinary approach is seen as crucial to the development of health care in the UK. 'Nurses, midwives, health visitors and the professions allied to medicine have long since taken the lead in providing effective and flexible solutions to changing patient needs, medical advances and shifts in the pattern of service delivery. They have expanded their scope for professional practice by developing in-depth specialist knowledge and skills in, for example, caring for patients with diabetes, glaucoma and mental illness' (Scottish Office 1997, p. 29). A similar acknowledgement is made for England and Wales (Department of Health 1997, p. 46).

The word 'professional' is normally used to describe a practitioner who has undergone a long course of training, the successful completion of which permits the candidate to be entered onto a register maintained by the ruling body of that profession. The professions are governed by statutes that legally support the ruling body of the profession and the regulation of practice. Examples of these statutes are the Professions Supplementary to Medicine Act 1960, the Nurses, Midwives and Health Visitors Act 1997 and the Osteopaths Act 1993. In the same way as any other legislation, these Acts may be amended, usually by the addition of Rules, to reflect changes in practice. Radical changes in the way in which nurses are trained has been given legal sanction by Rule 18 of the Nurses, Midwives and Health Visitors Act 1992, which lays out direction in the education and training of nursing students. It should be noted that this Act is currently under review.

Many professions that meet the sociological criteria of a profession are involved in health care delivery both in hospital and in the community. The largest group is formed by nurses and the therapy professionals – physiotherapists and occupational therapists – together with doctors. Other groups also make a significant contribution; pharmacists, including retail chemists, social workers and pastoral workers such as chaplains and counsellors are examples of these.

A Legal Framework for Caring

Thinking point

Think of one of the clients you are caring for. How many different groups are involved in his or her care?

Now think of your care group as a whole. List the different groups of professionals who may contribute to care delivery or who can be called on if necessary to support the client.

Many of the professionals you will have listed fulfil the formal criteria for a professional in that they have followed a course of training:

Traditionally, a professional person is associated with control of entry to a particular profession: the requirement to undergo a recognised length of training, accredited and, in some cases licensed, by an acknowledged professional body. (Leathard 1994, p. 6)

The training must also relate to the specific knowledge and practice of the profession. As modern health care becomes increasingly complex, extended or specialist roles may become a feature of the professional's work after basic training has been completed. The adoption of an extended or specialist role usually requires that further training may be undertaken, together with certification that the practitioner is competent to perform the role required; in some cases, further registration may be involved. An example of this is given by the prescription of drugs by midwives and nurses. Drug prescription is traditionally undertaken by a doctor; however, in clearly outlined circumstances, a midwife or a nurse with specific qualifications may prescribe drugs from a limited list. In order to do this, the practitioner has had to undertake further training and be registered as capable of meeting safe practice in this respect.

Professional behaviour is outlined in the codes or rules of professional conduct and ethics developed by the registering bodies. The behaviour expected of students of the profession is also included, as by the Chartered Society of Physiotherapy, or may, as adopted by the UKCC, take the form of a separate document. The significance of these documents cannot be underestimated as they form a standard of behaviour against which all members of the profession may be measured by an outsider, including a judge in court. The codes and rules, while they are not the law of the land in themselves, are closely rooted in the law. Practitioners who fall foul of the code of their registering body may find themselves being disciplined by a panel of their peers, with a consequent loss of registration and income. Professional disciplinary hearings are open to observation by members of that profession, and in addition, the results of disciplinary hearings are often published in the appropriate journals, although how the result was derived is not made public.

Analysis of the various codes and rules of conduct published by the professions shows much broad similarity. The codes cover the behaviour of the individual practitioner towards the client, behaviour towards the other members of the multidisciplinary team, behaviour towards students of the profession and integrity in commercial dealings where they are related to practice.

Client-centred behaviours emphasise the necessity of protecting the client, the maintenance of well-being and preservation of client safety at all times:

Each registered nurse, midwife and health visitor shall… act always in such a manner as to promote and safeguard the interests and well-being of patients and clients. (UKCC 1992, Clause 1)

A reflection on the increasing autonomy of all groups of non-medical professionals is an accent on the importance of gaining consent to treatment from the client: 'normally, every effort should be made to ensure that the client understands the nature, purpose and likely effect of the proposed treatment before being undertaken' (College of Occupational Therapists 1995, p. 6).

A common feature of such codes and rules is that professionals are bound to report to a superior when care cannot be delivered safely or when poor standards of care are experienced. This promotes health care professionals' position as the client's advocate in order to prevent risk to the individual for whom they are caring. The professional requirement to report unsafe circumstances to a superior supports the ideology of the Health and Safety at Work etc. Act 1974 whereby risks to either client or carer must be reported. A full written record of any instance of poor standards or unsafe practice should be made at the time of the incident.

The vital nature of the multidisciplinary team in the delivery of care is highlighted by the importance placed by the codes and rules on safe and effective collaboration with other members of the health care team and the client's relatives. Working with relatives may at times be controversial in that the client has a right to confidentiality and the client's wishes must be respected. In this situation, both professional experience and judgement may be required. The Chartered Society of Physiotherapists advises in Rule IV that 'Chartered physiotherapists shall communicate and co-operate with professional staff and other carers in the interests, and with the consent of their patient; and shall avoid criticism of any of them' (Chartered Society of Physiotherapists 1996, p. 2).

Dictionary definitions of the word 'profession' do not always agree in all respects, but the necessity for a distinct body of knowledge and a responsibility for the registered member both to maintain that knowledge and to pass it on to students of the profession are key features in all codes and rules of conduct. Indeed, it could be argued that professional knowledge of a suitable level must also be passed to unqualified staff in order to deliver quality care as demanded by the ruling bodies.

Thinking point

> Considering the members of the multidisciplinary team, do students of the professions work in the area where you are employed?
>
> How is the need for other, unqualified, staff met in terms of training?

The multidisciplinary approach is vital to the success of modern health care and the rehabilitation of elderly and disabled clients. Clients' physical, psychological and spiritual needs may be met by a variety of professionals in order to promote a successful outcome or the relief of distress. Each client will have his or her own needs, and co-ordination of the team is an important skill for the lead worker in health care.

Record-keeping

The importance and value of good records and record-keeping in health care cannot be overstated. What may seem a boring and routine task is of vital importance in the assessment of standards of care, in dealing with any complaints that may arise and for the support of staff in the event of legal action. Client-based records are confidential to the client and may contain sensitive information, so security of the records is also an important topic. Clients have a right of access to their own reports under two Acts of parliament: the Data Protection Act 1984 if the records are computerised, and the Access to Health Records Act 1990. Provided that access to these records is not considered by a medical practitioner to risk causing severe physical or mental distress, clients may access their own records, usually under the supervision of the doctor or dentist responsible for their care. It thus follows that records should be clearly written with the minimum use of technical jargon.

The client has a right of access to health care records under the Acts, but the principal use of health care records is to inform all workers of the client's treatment and care. The professional assessment of the client's needs is included, and a plan of care – decided upon whenever possible by both the health care professional and the client – is outlined. Importantly, an evaluation of the care, detailing what has been delivered to the client and by whom, is also integral to the overall record. In addition, the records will show which member of the multidisciplinary team delivered aspects of care and in which order the care, treatments or therapies were delivered. This is particularly vital when care is being delivered by more than one professional group; for example records held by nursing staff should acknowledge the contribution of therapy staff even though the therapy professionals hold their own records. In an attempt to simplify multidisciplinary record-keeping and facilitate audit, some clinical areas are now using shared record-keeping. This includes the contributions written by all the professional team, including records of case conferences with the details of everyday input.

Quality assurance in caring

At first sight, quality assurance and the development of standards of care that may be audited seem difficult to achieve in health care. Despite the fact that there is little legal basis for this area of practice, it does have important connotations for the handling of complaints and the increasing levels of litigation under civil proceedings that question poor or bad care delivery. There is also an ethical requirement to deliver the highest possible level of care to each client.

Quality assurance is the measurement of the actual level of the service provided plus the efforts to modify, when necessary, the provision of those services in the light of the results of measurement. (Sale 1996, p. 39)

The care of one client may involve many different professional groups, all of whom have their own input to the individual client's progress. Standards of care may be devised either on a unidisciplinary basis – for example, nursing – which reflects the contribution made by other professional groups, or on a multidisciplinary approach, which gives equal weight to all those involved. The multidisciplinary form of standards does, however, require a great deal of co-ordination and collaboration between each group and in practice can be complex. Ideally, standards of care are developed by practitioners working within a particular setting, and examine all aspects of care through assessment, planning, delivery and documentation. The practitioners, usually one or more registered professionals, are the people most likely to be fully aware of current developments in practice and the professional requirements that they must achieve. The standard, once developed, must have measurable outcomes that can be verified through an audit process by a third party. The adoption of this approach to care allows the monitoring of care delivery and an easy recognition of success or an early warning when matters are less than satisfactory.

When it goes wrong – whistleblowing

Whistleblowing has been defined as:

The unauthorised disclosure of information that an employee reasonably believes evidences the contravention of any law, rule or regulation, code of practice, or professional statement, or that involves mismanagement, corruption, abuse of authority, or danger to public or worker health and safety. (Vinten 1994, p. 257)

Vinten's definition essentially describes a breach in the duty of care that is legally owed by health care workers to those in their care, or to management issues that make it difficult or impossible to deliver care safely. Legal action for breach of the duty of care may range from the involvement of civil law to outright criminal proceedings being taken for a breach of criminal law following investigation by the police in serious instances.

Staff who observe an incident that they feel may be unacceptable, in that there is a risk to either the client or themselves and other carers, should report it immediately to their manager, making a documentary record of the incident. Professional students should also discuss the matter with their college. Students are often in a very difficult position in that they are 'passing through' on a placement and may later wish to seek employment in that, or a similar, area of practice. A further source of guidance and support for a person who feels that clients or staff are being placed at risk through malpractice may be gained from trade unions and professional organisations, some of whom, in order to support their members, have developed guidelines on whistleblowing and the correct procedure to adopt.

Whistleblowing is a complex issue, involving practitioners for whom bad practice may have unthinkingly become the norm, managers who have to make ends meet, clients and those who are trusted with their care. Needless to say, it has the potential to make the staff member very unpopular with the employer, so should only follow careful investigation of all the circumstances prior to reporting. In order to protect the client, professional codes place registered practitioners under a duty to report bad practice, with little protection for them should they do so. Students of the professions are placed in an even more difficult position; although they can be supported by their college, the necessity to find employment at the end of their course may affect their willingness to report breaches in the duty of care owed by health care workers to those in their charge.

Complaints

Publication of the *Patient's Charter* in 1992 (Department of Health 1992), to be superseded by the promised NHS Charter, gives clients stated expectations of NHS care delivery. Allied to an increasing will on the part of the public to complain and to resort to legal action if necessary, all health workers should have a knowledge of how to handle complaints as and when they arise. It is logical that, if a potential complaint can be avoided in its very early stages, less distress will be caused to the client, the carers and also the health care workers. The Hospital Complaints Procedure Act 1985, and subsequent guidelines from the DoH (1995) that became effective in 1996, ensures that the NHS has structures and policies to respond actively to the complainant. Evidence of auditable standards of care, codified professional behaviours and policies are helpful in the resolution of complaints. Within the NHS, it is a requirement to have a policy, with which all staff must be familiar, on the handling of complaints.

Thinking point

> If you work within the NHS, in any capacity, find out the following:
>
> What is the locally agreed policy on handling complaints?
>
> If a client, or carer, wishes to make a complaint, what procedure should he or she follow?

The complaint will, hopefully, be resolved at local level. Occasionally, those making the complaint feel that they have not been fairly treated, because of maladministration of the complaints procedure, or that the complaint has not been fully resolved. In this situation, they may appeal to the Health Service Commissioner – the Ombudsman – whose activities are outlined in the Health Service Commission Act 1993. An approach can only be made to the Ombudsman once all local procedures have been exhausted and the complaint has been subject to examination by an independent review. Each year, the total number of cases referred to the Ombudsman's office rises: 'The total number of complaints received in 1997–98 was 2,660, an increase of 20 per cent over 1996–97' (Health Service Commissioner 1998, Para 4.3).

While complaints and their treatment within the NHS are clearly structured, the position in the private sector is less clear. The person making the complaint should first approach the manager or officer in charge of care provision. If, at this stage, the complaint cannot be resolved, it may be that the person who feels aggrieved will have to approach the local authority if a registered home is implicated. A fuller discussion on the registration procedure relating to registered homes is given in Chapter 5. Other alternatives are to have recourse to legal action and to sue for redress.

Research ethics

Research is an important aspect of professionalism and, within health care, has traditionally been conducted by doctors. Rising academic standards among other health care professionals have meant that other professional groups are increasingly conducting research projects as part of either their education or their normal work. Other less formal research projects might be conducted in the workplace, for example the testing of a new approach to care by a particular staff group, or the investigation of a topic of interest to the health care team. In all cases, members of the care team may become involved in the project either on the fringes of the research or, in some cases, as participants. Research is principally conducted to enhance care and relies on several principles, one of which is beneficence (see above): 'The principle of beneficence requires that health care professionals engaged in research act to promote the well-being and benefit of participants' (Singleton and McLaren 1995, p. 118). This important principle is supported by the professional codes, all of which emphatically insist that the well-being of the client is paramount for the registered practitioners.

A further central principle of research in any field is that of non-maleficence, which, although closely related to beneficence, relates to any harm that might occur. This includes ensuring that workers engaged in research projects are properly qualified and supervised. If there is a risk of physical or psychological harm, all efforts must be made to minimise distress. Close liaison with an ethics committee needs to form an essential feature of the planning stages of any project involving clients: 'It is incumbent on research workers and ethical committees to ascertain that the safeguards which ensure harm does not occur are securely in place' (Singleton and McLaren 1995, p. 119).

The third major principle in research ethics is that of participant autonomy. This relates not so much to the researcher as to those who are taking part in the research project as the sample. Informed consent in care is used to describe the weighing of benefit against risk before treatment is commenced. In clinical research situations, the same principle holds true: 'It is imperative that potential subjects are warned of the potential risks of involvement before they agree to participate' (McHaffie 1996, p. 31). Risk, it must be reiterated, may involve either physical or psychological factors, and the management of foreseen risk could include such tactics as arranging for counselling to be available. Informed consent also normally includes an assurance of confidentiality. However, this can present the researcher with a dilemma should bad practices be revealed during the course of the project.

Ethical clearance for research in the NHS, and for research projects being conducted locally, is given by the local research ethics committee, a body set up by the local health authority to examine proposed research together with any associated ethical difficulties. The research project may only take place once clearance has been given by the committee and permission granted for the research project to start. Membership of the local research ethics committee normally involves representatives of the major professions involved in health care delivery – medicine, nursing and the therapy professions – together with laymen such as religious leaders, and local NHS Trust non-executive members. Professional representatives are deemed to be giving (or refusing) approval on behalf of their peers. The committee considers research projects of all types, for example drug trials and research projects involving clients, as well as any matter that has a major ethical slant.

Conclusion

This chapter has introduced many of the issues facing health care professionals, professional students and health care workers in practice today. The structure of the largest health care provider – the NHS – has been considered, together with the ways in which public opinion can influence the development of the NHS as a provider of health care in the future. Terms and conditions of employment have also been examined, as has the part played by trade unions in health care. Additionally, professional frameworks, as exemplified by codes and rules of conduct, have also been introduced. All health care professionals, together with their students, should be familiar with these essential documents, which, despite not forming part of the body of the law, underpin professional practice and may be used as a yardstick against which to measure that practice.

The importance of the maintenance of full, accurate records cannot be ignored as a basic legal requirement of practice and in order to provide evidence of the care that has been delivered. The length of time that it can take between a complaint being made and its resolution, or in the event of legal proceedings, renders memory unreliable, leaving only the evidence of records made at the time.

Quality assurance in health care is an important part of maintaining high standards of care and of the increasingly important audit that highlights the success or failure of approaches and strategies in care delivery. Sadly, sometimes not all goes well, and complaints may arise either within the system, from its own employees in the shape of whistleblowing, or from its consumers in the form of official complaints about health care.

Research is a feature of modern health care, and research matters may touch many who work with clients. All health care workers need to be familiar with the legal and ethical issues that surround them in this respect; in this chapter, only the professional focus has been examined. Informed consent by a client is examined more fully in the relevant chapters of this work, the broad issues of consent to treatment being equally applicable to their inclusion in a research project.

References and further reading

Chartered Society of Physiotherapists (1996) *Rules of Professional Conduct.* London, Chartered Society of Physiotherapists

College of Occupational Therapists (1995) *Code of Ethics and Professional Conduct for Occupational Therapists.* London, College of Occupational Therapists

Department of Health (1992) *The Patient's Charter.* London, HMSO

Department of Health (1995) *Government Response to Review of NHS Complaints Procedures Incorporating Acting on Complaints. EL(95)37.* London, HMSO

Department of Health (1997) *The New NHS: Modern, Dependable.* London, HMSO

Ham C (1997) *Health Care Reform, Learning from International Experience.* Buckingham, Open University Press

Health Care Financial Management Association (1995) *Introductory Guide to NHS Finance in the UK* (3rd edn). London, HFM/CIPFA

Health Service Commissioner (1998) *Health Service Commissioner – Fifth Report Session 1997–1998.* www.health.ombudsman.org.uk/hsc/document/hc811/chap-4.htm.

House of Commons Social Services Committee (1984) *Griffiths NHS Management Inquiry Report.* London, HMSO

Keenan D (1995) *Smith and Keenan's English Law* (11th edn). London, Pitman

Leathard A (ed.) (1994) *Going Inter-professional: Working Together for Health and Welfare.* London, Routledge

Lockton D (1994) *Employment Law.* Basingstoke, Macmillan

McHaffie H (1996) Ethical Issues in Nursing Research. In Cormack DFS (ed.) *The Research Process in Nursing* (3rd edn). Oxford, Blackwell Science, pp. 30–9

McHale J (1998) The Nurse and the Legal Environment. In McHale J, Tingle J and Peysner J (eds) *Law and Nursing.* Oxford, Butterworth Heinemann, pp. 1–15

Marshall E (1995) *General Principles of Scots Law* (6th edn). Edinburgh, W Green/Sweet & Maxwell

Sale D (1996) *Quality Assurance for Nurses and Other Members of the Health Care Team* (2nd edn). Basingstoke, Macmillan

Scottish Office (1997) *Designed to Care: Renewing the National Health Service in Scotland.* Edinburgh, Stationery Office

Singleton J and McLaren S (1995) *Ethical Foundations of Health Care.* London, CV Mosby

UKCC (1992) *Code of Professional Conduct.* London, United Kingdom Central Council for Nursing, Midwifery and Health Visiting

UKCC (1993) *Midwives Rules.* London, United Kingdom Central Council for Nursing, Midwifery and Health Visiting

Vinten G (1994) Whistle while you work in the health-related professions? *Journal of the Royal Society of Health*, October: 256–62

Webster G (1988) *The Health Services since the War* (vol. 1) Chapter 2. London, HMSO

Chapter 3 Working with the client

Introduction

Working with people within the health care setting may provoke, at times, conflict and debate as different moral and ethical viewpoints are involved in the delivery of care. Clients of the health care services may hold very different views of what is right or wrong compared with those held by the providers of the services. Members of the health care team may also hold different opinions on how correct treatment and care should be delivered to the individual clients.

Some of the issues discussed in this chapter are broadly those which are covered by professional codes and rules of conduct but may also be included in contracts of employment. For example, confidentiality is a major concern within health care provision. For concerns such as confidentiality, there is little legal basis for the client except for possible redress through civil law – the main control over health care workers in this case being via the contract of employment and proceedings through industrial relations mechanisms. Topics such as accountability are a vital feature of a health care professional's work and are a professional and management issue as opposed to one of legal action through the courts. Care is the central core of client provision; this chapter examines the duty of care to clients and its legal basis, together with its antithesis – negligence. Many of those admitted to full-time health care have altered mental processes that render them liable to confusional states and in some cases violent outbursts. Restraining clients may be necessary for their own safety and that of others around them. Restraint and false imprisonment are considered in the chapter.

Health care workers are individuals and may sometimes be involved in matters that are deeply distasteful to them. The legal position with regard to conscientious objection is considered, together with the ways in which health care professionals and workers can make their objections known.

Confidentiality

Just as it is difficult in our own lives to trust a friend who is likely to gossip, clients must be able to trust health care workers who hold personal information about them. Confidentiality and the treatment of a client's personal information are central to health care by all professional groups. Information regarding clients cannot be freely disclosed to any third party without the client's express consent to do so. Despite this important principle, there is no direct legislation requiring that the health care worker, professional or otherwise, maintain the confidentiality of client information. The importance of client trust and the confidentiality of personal information is first acknowledged in many cases by the contract of employment signed when a worker commences employment in the health care sector. The majority of contracts – including those signed by agency staff and honorary contracts signed by students – contain a confidentiality clause placing restraints on what information about clients in their care may be given and to whom. Large employers, such as hospitals, will also have published policies to give directions to staff. Action could therefore be taken against the individual worker through industrial relations legislation with the ultimate consequence of loss of employment. Registered professionals are covered by their codes and rules of conduct, thus also placing their registration in jeopardy should they be found guilty of breaking confidence, except in certain rare circumstances.

Common law (Scottish delict) is a potential source of reparation for the client by means of an injunction to prevent disclosure, or by suing the individual health worker for damages. However, Finch (1994, p. 391) advises that:

The courts might find that the medical practitioner's obligation not to disclose anything about his patient or his patient's affairs save on proper occasion was a legal duty no less than a moral obligation and may give a remedy (damages or injunction, or both) to a patient who had suffered loss or damage to reputation, or even embarrassment, as a result of a breach of that duty. But there has so far been no such decision, and any such legal action would be highly speculative.

Legislation does, however, exist to prevent the unauthorised disclosure of client information rather than its confidentiality as such. The Data Protection Act 1984 refers to information held on computer about an individual. The Act is not primarily aimed at health care but applies to all those who have personal details held on a computer. It does though have immense relevance for health care. The Data Protection Act 1984 has eight main principles, of which the eighth is particularly directed at security of information:

8. Appropriate security measures shall be taken against unauthorised access to, or alteration, disclosure or destruction of, personal data and against accidental loss or destruction of personal data. (Darley *et al.* 1994, p. 10)

Although the Data Protection Act does not apply to clients who have died, both contractual restraints and the professional codes and rules retain force following the client's death. Many client records are not held on computer, either because they pre-date computerisation or because records are held in a handwritten form. The Access to Medical Reports Act 1988 allows clients access to medical reports written about them at the request of a third party, for example for insurance purposes or prior to employment. Although the report is normally requested by the insurance company, mortgage provider or employer, the client has to consent to the report being compiled and to the information being disclosed to the third party. There are time limits to the client's action, and if he or she wishes the information to be kept from the organisation requesting it, this must be requested either at the time of the report or before it is supplied. The Access to Health Records Act 1990 covers very similar ground to the Data Protection Act 1984 but applies to written records; it does, however, only cover health records made since November 1991 when the Act was implemented. The Act gives the patient, or the authorised agent, a right of access to health records.

The disclosure of personal information about a client is therefore a prime concern of all those who work with clients who, by definition, are vulnerable and open to abuse of their confidential information. Information nevertheless needs to be shared between health care workers, or else the multidisciplinary team working for the client's benefit could be considerably handicapped. Students within the health care professions also need to exchange information in order to develop their skill and expertise in given situations. The rules and codes of conduct of the professional bodies include clauses permitting the sharing of information with others concerned in client care providing that it is in strict professional confidence. Once again, public disclosure is forbidden by the use of contracts of employment and potential disciplinary proceedings.

Rules regarding the disclosure of confidential information are easily breached unintentionally. In a process described as 'inappropriate comments', Ubel *et al.* (1995) examined conversations taking place in public places, including the lifts in a public hospital. Conversations taking place on public transport, in restaurants and in other public places can easily be overheard by passers-by who may, or may not, be related to or involved with the client under discussion. Admittedly, many comical and indeed sad things do happen to clients, but discussing them in a public place is a breach of their confidentiality and needs to be treated seriously.

Thinking point

Think of your own experience. Have you heard health care workers making 'inappropriate comments' in a public place. Public places include lifts, restaurants and any other areas to which the general public have access.

Sharing confidential information is sometimes necessary, even condoned by law, to impart confidential information to others. At its simplest, consent to disclose the information to a named third party is gained from the client and may then be imparted without breaching the client's rights in the matter. Another simple case concerns how much statistical evidence is drawn from causes of death or illness. The trends, once analysed, can inform governmental policy and shape advice given to the public regarding their health. This information is compiled with the client remaining anonymous, so no breach of the ethics of confidentiality is involved.

The importance of family involvement, or that of close friends, is often closely related to the care of the client, but what of the client's right to privacy? Korgaonkar and Tribe (1995, p. 144), discussing disclosure, suggest that:

Consent to disclosure may, however, also be implied so that, for example, while a patient may not have given express consent to the nurse to impart information about his condition to the next of kin, the right to do this would be implied unless instructions had been given to the contrary.

The concept of disclosure to next of kin is particularly important in the case of children when the parent or guardian is closely involved with the welfare of the child receiving treatment or care. Health care workers can face difficulties, however, when the complexity of modern family life is involved. How much should the partner of the child's parent be told? In the care of the elderly, where four-generation families are not uncommon, how many relatives should be involved in giving information? The next of kin is normally therefore included within the broad ethics governing confidential information and its disclosure, with them acting as a channel of information for the rest of the family.

There are situations when health care professionals have to consider other possibilities – a worried relative or friend enquiring after the client's welfare over the telephone – or occasions when confidential information might be transmitted using a fax machine. Telephone enquiries are a difficult matter to resolve unless the next of kin is well known to the care staff. While telephone banking is well established, together with checks on the caller's status, it is far more difficult to verify the caller's right to information over the telephone. In this situation, only generalised information should be given unless the care worker replying is certain of the caller's identity.

There are, however, clearly delineated situations when disclosure in the public interest is permissible and is indeed a statutory requirement. The Public Health (Control of Disease) Act 1984 requires a doctor to notify the District Medical Officer of certain infectious diseases outlined within the Act or its Regulations. Other statutes under which the doctor has to notify involvement relate to birth and death, as such anonymised information forms part of national statistics as covered by the NHS Notification of Births and Deaths Regulations 1974. The Abortion Act 1967 requires a doctor to notify the termination, the information – anonymised – again forming a national statistic. The other major area of disclosure is in drug addiction where, under the Misuse of Drugs Act 1971 (1973 Regulations), a doctor is required to notify the Home Office Chief Medical Officer that a client is being treated for addiction to specific drugs, examples being heroin and cocaine.

Care staff of all professions may occasionally be faced with the ethical decision of whether to disclose confidential information regarding the abuse of those in their care to social services or the police. Particularly in the case of adult abuse, this may be a matter of considerable difficulty, as many abused elderly people are afraid that, should abuse come to the notice of the authorities, they may lose either their home or contact with their relatives. In child abuse, if 'a registered practitioner has reason to suspect child abuse, he will have an ethical obligation to volunteer information to an appropriate authority, such as Social Services' (Schutte 1996, p. 65). At the present time in the UK, there is no legal obligation to notify an appropriate authority, although in some states of the USA and Australia, it is a legal requirement to report the abuse. In these legislatures, the care and treatment of the abused person, whether child or adult, is paramount, and rights to confidentiality and to disclosure are withdrawn in such cases, informants being immune from any form of legal action providing the information they give is in good faith. Within these legal systems both child and dependent adult abuse are given equal weighting.

The position held by the police is clear: 'Neither a nurse or doctor has any legal obligation to divulge confidential information to the police' (Korgaonkar and Tribe 1995, p. 146), although, under the Road Traffic Act 1988, anybody, when requested by the police, must give the name and address of a driver if an injury has, or is suspected to have, been suffered in an accident or if there is reason to believe that an offence has been committed under the Act. Only the name and address may be given, and no clinical or other details should be divulged.

Confidentiality and the related disclosure of personal information are of vital importance to all grades of staff and all professions in the health care sector. Emphasis is placed on the maintenance of confidentiality by contracts of employment and by the codes of conduct and rules of all the professional bodies involved in client care. Only in a few clearly outlined cases is disclosure condoned by the law, these being contained in, and outlined by, orders of court.

Duty of care and accountability/responsibility

The duty of care is an important concept in the provision of health care by one person to another. Young (1995, p. 13) defines the duty of care thus: 'A person must take reasonable care to avoid acts or omissions that he can reasonably foresee would be likely to injure a person directly affected by those acts.' Clients coming into contact with health care workers have a right to the best treatment and care available to them and may have recourse to the law via either civil or, in the case of for example assault, criminal law. The English duty of care is closely linked to the Scottish categories of rights and obligations: 'In law, obligations go hand in hand with rights; if one party is under an obligation, then some other party has a corresponding right' (Marshall 1995, p. 298). Within both legal systems, the matter is greatly simplified if a written contract exists, but this is unlikely in the situation of health care. How then may the duty of care be assessed in law?

Health care workers can be broadly divided into three groups. The first group comprises registered professionals, whose registering bodies have produced a document outlining the duties of those registered with them by the means of a code or rules of conduct for the profession. This document will enable a judge to decide whether or not the professional was acting within the expectations of the professional body. Second come students studying for entry to the register of their profession. In some cases, the registering body has produced a code or rules specifically for students of the profession. However, students are normally deemed to be working under the supervision of the registered member and are basically not liable for their actions. Despite this, the actions expected of a senior student in the immediate pre-registration stage would reasonably be close to those of a newly qualified member. The third group is that of unqualified staff who, while not liable to a professional body, still have a basic duty of care to their clients, normally within the expectations of their job.

Accountability for the actions taken in the delivery of care to clients is an important professional concept:

Accountability is not a word that is used within a legal context but is important professionally. Definitions usually emphasize responsibility for actions, being answerable and making decisions based on knowledge and understanding. Legally it is therefore a concept closely related to that of duty of care and negligence. (Young 1995, p. 17)

Professional codes and rules stipulate that professionals are accountable for the actions that they take as well as their omissions, so they may be responsible to a number of bodies for these actions. For example, a professional is likely to be responsible to the employer, the professional body and potentially, through civil law, to the patients themselves. Nor should it be overlooked that all groups in health care are accountable to themselves – it may be very difficult to live with some action that has caused harm or unnecessary distress to a client. Particularly within nursing, the extended role whereby a nurse undertakes duties formerly done by others, frequently medical practitioners, is a feature of care delivery and this situation is covered by the code of conduct. The UKCC document *The Scope of Professional Practice* advises practitioners that they 'must acknowledge any limits of personal knowledge and skill and take steps to remedy any relevant deficits in order effectively and appropriately to meet the needs of patients and clients' (UKCC 1992, p. 6). In many cases, employers have developed training programmes for these extended roles in order to ensure good practice by the individual practitioner. Other professional bodies, for example the Chartered Society of Physiotherapists, cover the actions of independent practitioners, whose practice has to be covered by insurance as they may be individually accountable to civil law for their practice. Importantly, it is a feature of all the codes that it is unacceptable for professionals to act outside their expertise.

Mechanisms are available by which the behaviour, and therefore the accountability, of care providers may be measured. The contract of employment, usually allied to a job description, outlines what duties are expected of the employee and will be written to relate to either registered or unqualified workers. The job description will then state more clearly the expectations in behaviour and practice, and also to whom the individual is accountable for management purposes. Students of the professions will find that the course documents outline the expected level of practice pertinent to their progression on the course, and that the training body will demand some form of accountability from them, usually by means of the successful completion of both practice and theoretical assignments.

Accountability and responsibility are closely linked; care staff may be responsible for their actions and accountable to either management or their profession for those actions.

Thinking point

The head of home in a small residential facility in the community decides that the clients would benefit from an outing. The head asks Angela, a senior care assistant, to take charge of the arrangements.

Who is responsible for the arrangements being made?

To whom will they be accountable?

Negligence

Duty of care, accountability and responsibility are very closely linked if a client wishes to sue for negligence. It is important to stress here that, in civil law in England and delict in Scotland, it is the clients or their representatives who must prove the wrong. Montgomery (1995, p. 80) sums up the English situation if a case of negligence is to be proved: 'Was the professional responsible for the patient? Did she fail in her responsibility? Did her failure injure the patient?' The Scottish system is broadly similar in that a duty of care to the client must exist, the standard of care is that expected of the practitioner, and there is proof of the negligence. Marshall (1995, p. 505) does, however, make the observation that 'During the course of the case, however, the evidence may have the effect of shifting the onus of proof on to the defender, with the result that it will be for the defender to prove that he has not been negligent, if he is to escape liability for delict', and this situation is equally liable to exist within the English legal system. Again, it can be seen that a clear outline of the duties and standards expected of health care workers, both professionally registered and otherwise, is in the interests of both the worker and the employer, who is likely to be taking liability for the actions of the employee. The certification of higher skills is also important as proof that the practitioner has been trained and is able to perform the skill safely. Once practitioners have been trained, and should they then perform the skill carelessly, they could be found personally liable for any action taken against them. Similarly, if they have not undertaken the higher training and perform the task, they are also likely to be held liable. The standard legal test when skill is being judged is the 'Bolam test', derived from a ruling by the judge in a case against a hospital management committee:

The test is the standard of the ordinary skilled man exercising and professing to have that special skill. A man need not possess the highest expert skill at the risk of being found negligent. It is a well-established law that it is sufficient if he exercises the ordinary skill of an ordinary man exercising that particular art. (cited in Mason and McCall Smith 1994, p. 199)

In order to prevent harm to the client, the rules and codes of conduct clearly identify the right of their registered practitioners – and students where a code exists for them – to opt out of undertaking tasks for which they have not been properly trained or if they feel incapable of performing the task for any reason.

Negligence is an area in which the maintenance of good records in a written or retrievable form is absolutely vital. No health care worker can foresee all eventualities, the outcome of treatment or the side-effects of particular drugs as every client is an individual and needs to be treated as such. Legal action may take many years to come to fruition, by which time memories have faded and many will have moved to other employment. The importance of an accurate record made at the time is then invaluable if the practitioner is to defend an allegation of negligence within either the English or the Scottish legal system. In the absence of contemporary records, a court must assume that no action was taken as there is no proof that the action did in fact exist. The same applies to hearings before professional bodies. The finding of proof of negligence in court is likely to result in the registered practitioner being accountable to a professional body, with potential loss of registration and therefore employment.

Vicarious liability

The actions of an employed practitioner are normally protected by the principle of vicarious liability. In accepting vicarious liability, the employer takes responsibility for the actions of the employee provided that they are taken in the course of normal employment and not outside the worker's expected duties. The employer must insure against the actions of his employee in respect of any damage or injury the employee might cause to another worker under the Employer's Liability (Compulsory Insurance) Act 1969, and this is generally extended to cover the employee's activities towards clients, with the provision that the employee is acting within his or her normal expected duties. One major exception to this rule within health care is the situation of doctors working in the NHS, who, as they are permitted to act privately in addition to their NHS work, take partial responsibility for their professional actions and are accordingly responsible for insuring their practice. It is important to stress that the notion of vicarious liability extends to health care workers within their normal employment, as specified in the contract of employment and job description/specification if one is in existence. If health care workers are acting outside their employment, they accept personal liability if things go wrong. Trade union members are better protected than non-union members, as union membership often includes an element of professional indemnity cover for the member. Professional indemnity insurance covers the practitioners' professional duty with the provision that they are competent and qualified to undertake the duties. Independent practitioners may need to make their own indemnity arrangements, or alternatively membership of their professional body may include insurance cover.

Restraint and false imprisonment

Working with clients who are confused or who have a poor understanding of their situation and surroundings presents a major challenge for those delivering care. Care workers have to consider how far they may go in assuring the safety of the client and those around them without infringing the civil liberties of the client who is confused. The use of restraint may take the form of either chemical, using prescribed drugs, or physical means. Physical restraint methods may include cot sides, chairs or wheelchairs with a tray that prevents the client getting out of the chair, or any other method that restricts movement. Ideally, clients should be able to move freely according to their wish, but the prevention of injury either to the client or others may be an important care problem. Purpose-built units caring for those who are mentally impaired may feature a safely enclosed area where clients can walk without risk to themselves. Clients living in the community pose particular problems if they are liable to wander close to roads and heavy traffic. Where practical, the use of baffle locks or alarmed doors may prove useful in both the home and the institutional setting, but they can be difficult in practice on a busy ward in a general hospital. Restraint may place health care workers in a position where they could become liable under tort – a civil wrong (see Chapter 1) – for false imprisonment. Jones (1996) discusses how, under this tort, the individual does not have to be confined or any force used, no damage to them needs to have occurred, but their freedom of movement has to have been affected and escape from restraint made difficult. Thus the tort of false imprisonment becomes an important feature of the civil liberties of the individual in institutionalised care. The client need not be fully conscious for his or her rights to be infringed; as Stanton (1994) observes, 'conduct in breach of a person's rights is no less obnoxious because the victim is unconscious, asleep or in ignorance of what is happening'.

Many NHS Trusts and larger care employers have developed guidelines for the control and restraint of clients outlining which techniques are acceptable. These are particularly valuable in conjunction with staff training in the control of violent outbursts by clients.

Legal redress for restraint ranges from complaints made by either the client or the relatives to civil action under tort for false imprisonment or trespass to the person or even criminal proceedings for assault and battery. All health care staff should be extremely careful to maintain good, adequate and clearly written records of any incidents where restraint has been used to pacify clients or to ensure their safety as litigation may take many years to come to fruition.

Assault and battery/consent to treatment

In this section, the use of the words 'assault' and 'battery' are also used to cover the Scottish legal term 'assault'. In England, the modern law of trespass has evolved from medieval writs involving obstruction (or trespass) to the owner's land, goods or indeed person. Scottish law contains the category of 'delict', which concerns injury to the person covering similar broad ground to that of the English pattern. The two have been considered together in this section.

The original medieval law of trespass has evolved, and modern legal practice has further defined this to mean assault, battery and false imprisonment. All these three categories of trespass on the person may involve either civil action under tort or criminal proceedings. False imprisonment, particularly in the use of restraint, has been discussed in the previous section. Assault and battery may be a feature in the control and restraint of violent outbursts or a result of deliberate action or potential action to harm the client. Assault and battery are also clearly involved in the abuse of clients of whatever age, and occasionally – usually in cases well publicised by the media – a health care worker is accused of assault and battery. However, it should be recognised that the health care worker also has redress under the law for assault and battery by clients or their relatives, this is currently extremely rare but is a potential source of litigation.

The two terms, 'assault' and 'battery', are often used together but have distinct separate legal meanings and need not necessarily be linked together in court proceedings. Assault is the threat of force being used, whether imminently or in the future, while battery is the actual use of violence or force on a person. Health care workers who specialise in caring for clients who may be unpredictable and violent will often face threats of violence and actual physical risks, so training in the management and handling of violent incidents is important.

Assault and battery are relevant legal categories, not only in the clear-cut situation of violence, but also in areas where treatment is being carried out.

Consent by a client to a procedure removes the threat of action being taken against the professional who is carrying out the procedure: 'In the case of a competent adult patient any medical diagnosis or treatment which involves a direct application of force to the patient performed without the consent of the patient constitutes a battery' (Jones 1996, p. 417). Prior to surgery or many other procedures, it is necessary for the doctor performing the procedure to obtain consent from the patient, and the signed consent will be checked several times by different health care workers as part of the pre-operative preparation. The argument over informed consent and the patient's full understanding of the procedure and its outcome or effects forms part of an ongoing legal and ethical debate among professionals in the health care sector. An important point is that the professional performing the procedure in the mistaken belief that the patient had consented when in fact he or she had not is at risk of litigation, with those who act as double-checkers being liable to disciplinary proceedings by the employer. It is for this reason that stringent checking of documentation is vital before a patient is to undergo surgery or other invasive procedure. Consent may also be implied for minor procedures, for example the patient who extends an arm prior to a blood test indicating that he or she is willing for the blood to be taken. Increasingly, the guidelines used by other members of the multidisciplinary team require that the professional, or student, explain the procedure to patients in order that they may understand what is being done. There is also a responsibility to assess the client's understanding of the planned procedure in order to obtain valid consent.

Thinking point

> If you work in an area where patients/clients undergo invasive procedures, check how and when their consent is obtained and whether it is written consent.

Occasionally, consent may not be obtainable: an unconscious accident victim requiring immediate surgery to save life cannot give consent to surgery even if mutilating surgery is required. The argument of necessity is a defence against battery in such cases when the victim's life is at risk.

Consent to treatment raises the question of how consent may be obtained from those who are not mentally competent to give their agreement to a procedure. This group includes young children and clients of all ages whose mental state renders them unable to understand the implications of procedures. In these cases, the practitioner must be careful to follow established guidelines and legal precedents before the procedure is undertaken. In this situation, the practitioner needs carefully to assess the client's capability and understanding of the procedure. The legal and moral duty of care that is owed to vulnerable clients by those entrusted with their care is of vital importance and must not be overlooked.

Conscientious objection

The delivery of health care is full of moral and ethical dilemmas, and these may result in conflict between the client and health care workers. All parties will bring their personal beliefs and standards to decision-making about care, although it must always be borne in mind that the health care worker has a duty of care to the client by virtue of the position held by the worker. The opposite is not true; the patient owes no duty of care (or of accepting care) to the health care providers. Clients always retain the right to refuse aspects of care, up to and including the right to make an advance directive (living will), which specifies in writing treatments to which they will or will not agree.

Registered and student nurses are advised by the UKCC, the registering body, that they must make known any conscientious objections that they have to the treatment being delivered. A conscientious objector is one who feels deeply that an action is morally wrong. In the case of students of the professions, conscientious objection can often be accommodated quite simply by either changing the work placement or transferring them to another area of the workplace where their beliefs are not as likely to be challenged. However, students are undertaking a course in order to follow their chosen profession and mere dislike of a client group does not form a conscientious objection.

The difficulty is not so easily resolved when registered practitioners are faced with this problem. The legal right to conscientious objection is contained only within the Abortion Act 1967 and the Human Fertilisation and Embryology Act 1990, which allow nurses (and midwives) the right to refuse to participate in procuring the abortion, that is, to take part in the actual procedure.

A similar situation could be considered as existing when caring for clients who are either extremely ill or very elderly. Whether to resuscitate, or not to resuscitate, whether to grant patients their expressed wish to die – short of euthanasia – is also a dilemma for many staff. The Law Commission, as part of its draft legislation on mental incapacity, which includes advance directives, considers that conscientious objection is not appropriate in this situation as basic nursing care or pain control may not be withdrawn. This recommendation is helpful, but all health care workers as well as nurses should make their feelings known to the immediate manager or supervisor of their workplace; this is especially important if it is their actions which are keeping the patient alive.

Therapy staff may also face difficult choices when dealing with clients. How far should potentially painful treatment be pursued towards the ultimate goal of restoring function? The *Rules of Professional Conduct* for physiotherapists and the *Code of Ethics and Professional Conduct* for occupational therapists advise that their members may not take part in any treatment that is actively harmful and that potentially painful therapies may only be undertaken providing the patient understands the treatment, consents to it and is left as pain free as possible following the treatment. Within this framework, the client does of course at all times retain the right, sanctioned by the professional bodies, to refuse treatment should they wish.

References and further reading

Clarkson C and Kealing H (1994) *Criminal Law: Text and Materials* (3rd edn). London, Sweet & Maxwell

Darley B, Griew A, McLoughlin K and Williams J (1994) *How To Keep a Clinical Confidence: A Summary of Law and Guidance on Maintaining the Patient's Privacy*. London, HMSO

Finch J (1994) *Speller's Law Relating to Hospitals* (7th edn). London, Chapman & Hall Medical

Jones M (1996) *Textbook on Torts* (5th edn). London, Blackstone Press

Korgaonkar G and Tribe D (1995) *Law for Nurses*. London, Cavendish Publishing

Law Commission (1995) *Mental Incapacity (Part V) Law Commission 231*. London, HMSO

Marshall E (1995) *General Principles of Scots Law* (6th edn). Edinburgh, W Green & Son

Mason J and McCall Smith R (1994) *Law and Medical Ethics* (4th edn). London, Butterworth

Montgomery J (1997) *Health Care Law*. Oxford, Oxford University Press

Montgomery J (1995) Negligence. In Tingle J and Cribb A (eds) *Nursing Law and Ethics*. Oxford, Blackwell Scientific, pp. 79–92

Schutte P (1996) Confidentiality. In Payne-James J, Dean P and Wall I (eds) *Medico-legal Essentials in Health Care*. Edinburgh, Churchill Livingstone

Stanton K (1994) *The Modern Law of Tort*. London, Sweet & Maxwell

Ubel P, Zell M, Miller D, Fischer G, Peters-Stefani D and Arnald R (1995) Elevator talk: observational study of inappropriate comments in a public space, *American Journal of Medicine*, **99**: 190–4

UKCC (1992) *The Scope of Professional Practice*. London, United Kingdom Central Council for Nursing, Midwifery and Health Visiting

Weller B (1997) *Baillière's Nurses' Dictionary* (22nd edn). London, Baillière Tindall

Young A (1995) The legal dimension. In Tingle J and Cribb A (eds) *Nursing Law and Ethics*. Oxford, Blackwell Scientific, pp. 3–20

Chapter 4 Caring safely

Introduction

'To care for someone is to supply protection and preservation' (Kitson *et al.* 1992, p. 30). The very word 'caring' implies that the client should come to no harm, whether in hospital or in any other residential setting. The preservation of the client's safety, and that of the health care workers delivering care, is a topic of major importance and as such is recognised by legislation.

The administration of drugs is included in this chapter to emphasise both the importance of drugs in much of modern health care and the ways in which the legal system controls the supply of therapeutic drugs and the safety of those to whom they are being administered.

The 1974 Health and Safety at Work etc. Act began a new era in workplace safety for both employers and employees, and this is discussed in relation to contemporary health care practice. Because of its importance in the well-being of both client and health care worker, UK legislation in this area is closely harmonised with that of the EC and forms a good example of how closely the two systems are now linked.

It is well established that many work-related injuries in health care are the result of poor moving and handling techniques. The importance of the legislation in this area cannot be underestimated, either in the prevention of injury to staff and client or in the provision of adequate equipment and training by the employer. Dangerous occurrences within the workplace, including incidents of injury in moving and handling, must be reported, and the method by which this is done is examined. Health care workers are occasionally in contact with potentially hazardous or harmful substances, and their control is also considered.

Finally, the chapter discusses a subject vital to the maintenance of good health: the provision of safe and wholesome food and the legislation that covers this important aspect of care.

The administration of drugs

The administration of drugs is an important aspect of health care. It is recognised that only limited groups of health care professionals and workers may be involved in the administration of drugs to clients, but the legal framework is of great importance to these groups. Unqualified staff may well play a part in the administration or observation of the client for side-effects, whether beneficial or otherwise, reporting these accordingly to the qualified staff on duty. Within the hospital service, student nurses, and operating department practitioners in particular, may play quite a large part in drug administration as part of their training. In the community, staff in residential and children's homes may also play a role in the administration of medications. It follows therefore that a knowledge of the law underpinning medicines is of use to these groups.

Three major statutes are associated with the supply, storage and administration of drugs: the Medicines Act 1968, the Misuse of Drugs Act 1971 and the Medicinal Products: Prescription by Nurses Act 1992.

The Medicines Act 1968 controls the development and licensing of drugs, together with how they may be supplied and sold to the public, the packing and labelling of medicinal products, the work of local chemists and the publication of the British pharmacopoeia. A pharmacopoeia is 'an authoritative publication that gives the standard formula and preparations of drugs used in a given country' (Weller 1997, p. 321). Supply and sale to the public are also detailed by the Act in the form of Regulations to Part 3 of the Act that can be altered periodically in the light of changing practice and demand. The Act governs medicines that must be prescribed by a practitioner – most commonly a doctor – but dentists, midwives and some nurses may also prescribe specified drugs from limited lists. The labelling of the drugs that must be prescribed by a practitioner shows a small 'PoM' – standing for prescription-only medicine – usually surrounded by a printed box to indicate the status of the contents under the Medicines Act. Other drugs, for example bottles of paracetamol, may be bought directly from chemists, but only under the supervision of a registered pharmacist. The Regulations to the Medicine Act 1968 cover pharmacy-only medicines, the labels of which are marked with a capital P surrounded by a box. The third grouping of medications within the Regulations concern the 'general sales list', in which unopened containers of specified drugs may be sold to the public not necessarily from a retail chemist or pharmacy. This includes the small quantities of paracetamol or aspirin that can be bought over the counter in supermarkets and petrol stations.

Thinking point

Under supervision from a registered practitioner, look at the drug prescription chart for one of your clients. Make a note of the drugs and refer to a text to discover the actions and interactions of the drugs prescribed.

Think of your own experience. Have you been to a chemist and bought a P category medication? The assistant will bring the sale to the attention of the duty pharmacist or will be unable to make the sale if no registered pharmacist is present.

Wherever medications are to be administered, the safe storage of drugs is of importance to prevent accidental overdose or the misuse of drugs by people other than those for whom they are intended. Within hospitals, all drugs are kept within locked containers. These may take the form of cupboards, drug trolleys or refrigerators, all of which should be kept locked. Additional security is required for those drugs described as controlled drugs. The keys to the locked containers are held by the registered nurse in charge of the ward or department, or by a designated deputy. The situation is not so simple within the residential home sector, although there is still responsibility for medications and their safe custody, and often for administration to residents within the home. Residential homes are covered within the useful document *The Administration and Control of Medicines in Residential and Children's Homes* published by the Royal Pharmaceutical Society of Great Britain (RPSGB; 1994), the registering body for pharmacists, which includes local chemists' shops. The RPSGB advises that 'great emphasis is laid on the desirability of residents retaining custody of their own medicines, wherever possible'. However, the rising age and increasing disability of many older people in residential care, or those who are unable to take responsibility for their own drug administration, means that this is not always possible to achieve. The guidelines then advise that 'All other medicines must be stored in a locked cupboard or trolley and kept in a room not generally accessible to residents or visitors to the home.' The Society also advises on the training of unqualified staff in relation to the administration of medicines to those resident within the home.

The Misuse of Drugs Act 1971 and its Schedules are concerned with those drugs which are potentially addictive and are likely to be abused; these particular drugs do, however, have immense therapeutic value particularly in the control of pain. They are generally described as 'controlled drugs', although the term 'dangerous drugs' is still occasionally heard, referring to the legislation that preceded the Misuse of Drugs Act 1971. As with many other statutes, the Act has Regulations, the 1973 Regulations, which permit the use of the scheduled drugs in medicine, and the 1985 Regulations, which amended the Schedule to include other drugs, principally barbiturates and some appetite suppressants. The Act also covers the storage of these groups of drugs. In hospitals and nursing homes, 'Controlled drugs are required to be stored in a separate locked cupboard constructed to prevent unauthorised access to the drugs. It is customary for this cupboard to be within another locked cupboard' (Downie *et al.* 1995, p. 344). The Act also lays out stringent procedures for the ordering and prescribing of controlled drugs.

In recent years, publicity has been given to the innovation of nurse prescribing, and to this end the Medicinal Products: Prescription by Nurses Act 1992 was passed. The Act allows certain registered general nurses to prescribe from a limited list, an up-to-date version of which is included in each copy of the *British National Formulary*. The legislation is currently under review as the situation of nurses of all registrations working within the community extends. Midwives are also permitted to prescribe from within a limited list of drugs whose use is beneficial during labour and childbirth. These drugs, including pethidine – a controlled drug – are locally agreed between consultant obstetricians and senior midwifery staff, and take the form of standing orders that may be amended from time to time. Increasingly within hospitals, senior registered nurses are administering drugs by the use of protocols. The protocol is drawn up by medical consultants in collaboration with the nurses concerned and allows nurses to administer prescribed drugs to clients in certain circumstances only. The formats for both protocols and the midwives' locally agreed list of drugs are similar and, with the exception of the client's name, must contain all other details that are given on a normal prescription for an individual client in order to meet the requirements of the Medicines Act 1968. The documents are also signed by the consultant and co-signed by representatives of the groups of midwives or nurses involved.

Health and safety at work

Legal attention has been paid to the conditions under which many workers are employed in this country since mid-nineteenth-century Acts sought to preserve the safety of the workforce in the mines, children working in factories and railway workers. The pattern of industry-specific legislation continued until the latter half of the twentieth century when, by the 1970s, 30 statutes and 500 additional Regulations to the parent Acts were law in Britain, each one referring to conditions in an identified industry. Despite this mass of legislation, many workers were not covered by legal safety measures, health care workers forming a large number of those left out. The origins of the 1974 Health and Safety at Work etc. Act lay with the government-appointed Robens Committee (House of Commons 1972), which reported in 1972. Broadly, the Committee's findings were that: there was too much law; its piecemeal development resulted in a poorly structured and complex framework; the existing law was aimed only at physical harm and ignored psychological aspects of safety at work; and finally, enforcement of existing legislation was difficult because of its fragmentation.

The thrust of the earlier laws was very much one of the preservation of the safety of the employee; however, two other twentieth-century pieces of legislation are worthy of note in the overall picture of workplace safety. The 1897 Workman's Compensation Act made it a duty of the employer to provide some maintenance when an employee had been injured during the course of employment, and the Act was later extended to cover claims for some industrial diseases. Compensation under the Act was, however, small, and there was no duty for the employee to prove negligence on the part of the employer for payment to be made. The employee could claim for employer negligence under the Act using either the criminal or civil pathway but not both. The Act was repealed in 1948 by the 1946 National Insurance (Industrial Injuries) Act as it entered the statute book. The new Act retained the principle of income maintenance, with the difference that the state rather than the employee paid the benefits through the social security system. Damages for negligence could still be claimed from the employer, but, following the 1989 Social Security Act, any monies paid by the state could be reclaimed from the damages payable. This situation continues in relation to the social security benefits payable following industrial accidents.

The 1974 Health and Safety at Work etc. Act in many cases repealed the older Acts, while others were phased out. The Act provides a framework for general health and safety issues in all workplaces and allows for the future introduction of specific Regulations as well as laying out the general duties of all those affected by the Act. Within the general duties outlined in the Act are those of both the employer and, for the first time, the employee, who is also seen to have responsibilities under the Act. The employer has a duty to protect workers and the general public or others affected by the work undertaken, while the employee has a duty to know of the hazards existing in the workplace. All parties are to be involved in the prevention of workplace hazards and risks to health and safety. The Act also places an accent on the need for training, instruction and supervision in order to prevent workplace hazards; an example of this is given in the following section on moving and handling.

Liability under the Health and Safety at Work etc. Act 1974 is principally under civil law, with penalties under criminal law being reserved for instances of extreme negligence leading to serious injury or death.

Moving and handling

Moving and handling, a common feature of caring for dependent clients, is an example of how EC law can be integrated into a member country's own legal system. The moving and handling of loads is recognised by European law to be hazardous to the health of the person – in any occupation – who is required to do this as part of their job. To reduce the toll of injury and disability to workers, a European Directive (90/269/EEC) was applied on the 1 January 1993, as Regulations to the Health and Safety at Work etc. Act 1974 and the Management of Health and Safety at Work Regulations 1992. A Directive is one of the sources of European law and is mandatory for member states. It is aimed at states rather than the individual and has to be further incorporated into the member state's own law. Further discussion on this point was given in Chapter 1. However, in the UK, health care Trusts are considered to be state organisations and are therefore subject to Directives whether or not the Directive has been absorbed into national law. 'Thus the NHS is obliged to comply with the provisions of Community law even before they have been fully incorporated into English law' (Montgomery 1997, p. 17). In practice, this can result in the NHS adopting new working practices before they have been developed within the private sector, an example being the moving and handling Regulations. This can result in confusion as staff transfer from one sector to another. In order to make individuals and non-state organisations subject to the Directive, the device of additional Regulations to an already existing Act, in this case the Health and Safety at Work etc. Act 1974, is used.

Other sources of European law are treaties, as in the Treaty of Rome by which the UK became a member state of the EC. A Regulation made by the European Council – a European Regulation – is 'binding in its entirety and directly applicable in all member states' (Jenkins 1995, p. 8). Marshall adds that European Regulations will also 'override any part of our national law which is contrary to them' (Marshall 1995, p. 114). The final source for the interpretation of European law is the European Court of Justice in Luxembourg, which can decide matters for individuals, governments and other institutions, and whose decision is binding.

The moving and handling of dependent clients by health care staff is a common feature of practice in many settings. Over many years, it has become evident that injury and disability to staff can be linked to poor practice and repeated actions, often in far from ideal surroundings. Nor can the toll on health care workers be entirely linked to the moving of clients alone.

In your workplace, what items are staff likely to have to move and handle?

Which other members of staff may be involved in the moving and handling of either clients or goods?

Spend a few minutes making a list of these; include clients if this is likely, and also other items such as stores.

When and why do they have to be moved? Could any other means be used to get them from one place to another?

Consider how often these items have to be moved.

Logan (1996, p. 22) gives the estimate 'that 80 000 nurses are off work with back problems each year and 3600 do not return to work', but the problem is not confined to nursing and allied professions. 'Ambulance crews undertaking routine patient transport or emergency and paramedic services face particular manual handling problems' (Health and Safety Advisory Committee 1992, p. 19). The cost of these injuries is high, not only in financial terms to the employer, but also in terms of lost employment and pain for the employee.

In order to reduce the injury rate within health care delivery, Directive 90/269/EEC enshrined within the Regulations of the Health and Safety at Work etc. Act 1974 establishes clear guidelines. Employers are required to make an assessment of the risks of manual handling faced by their staff or to delegate the assessment to people working within the organisation who may have a specialist knowledge of the hazards faced. Once the assessment has been completed, action may be needed to alter the layout of the workplace as well as to provide suitable moving and handling equipment for the tasks required in order to reduce the risks faced by staff. The Health and Safety at Work etc. Act does 'require employers to provide their employees with health and safety information and training. This should be supplemented as necessary with more specific information and training on manual handling injury risks and prevention as part of the steps to reduce risk required by Regulation 4 (1)(b)(ii) of the present Regulations' (Health and Safety Executive 1996, p. 32). It is important to stress that, under health and safety legislation, the individual employee is also liable for his or her own practice. Employees must also take steps to assess any manual handling operation and reduce potential risks by making the area as safe as possible, using the equipment provided by the employer for the task and attending training sessions.

Record-keeping is a fundamental aspect of manual handling. This is particularly vital in an area where injuries can be clearly identified as linked to manual handling and where a high level of risk is known to exist. Written records may clearly become essential during legal proceedings for compensation or when injury has occurred to the client during moving. Equally, good records can form a vital part of the assessment of individual clients and their particular needs in order to aid the safety of both client and staff.

Injuries sustained at work are considered to be sufficiently important for them to become part of the formal reporting system to the Health and Safety Executive, RIDDOR.

RIDDOR and COSHH

As the European Directive on the manual moving and handling of loads has shown, the accurate reporting of injuries and potential dangers is a vital source of and motivation for the development of legislation protecting the individual in the workplace. In order to simplify the reporting of all types of accident or danger in the workplace, a group of Regulations under the Health and Safety at Work etc. Act 1974 have been combined in the Reporting of Injuries, Diseases and Dangerous Occurrences Regulations 1995, which became law in April 1996. 'Reporting accidents and ill health at work is a legal requirement. The information enables the enforcing authorities to identify where and how risks arise and to investigate serious accidents' (Health and Safety Executive 1996, p. 1). The Regulations cover work-based injuries and diseases in several categories: death or major injury, disease related to the workplace, dangerous occurrences and 'over-3-day injuries'. This last group is likely to be the one into which injuries sustained during moving and handling fall. Should an employee – and employees may include students working with an honorary contract – be unfortunate enough to be included within the reportable categories, an accident report form needs to be sent 'to the enforcing authority within ten days' (Health and Safety Executive 1996, p. 3). Employers must keep records of reportable incidents either in written form or on a computer. Computerised records are subject to the Data Protection Act 1984, and the information held may only be disclosed to people authorised to receive the information. The RIDDOR Regulations also allow for the recognition of potential dangers – dangerous occurrences – even though no injury has occurred. This can identify faults in equipment or safety that may highlight defects in the manufacture of equipment or its use and allow for suitable safety measures to be taken.

The aim of contemporary health and safety legislation is to prevent accidents occurring, and while the RIDDOR Regulations allow for the reporting of potential hazards, another set of Regulations, those for the Control of Substances Hazardous to Health – COSHH – require that employers assess the risk of danger from any hazardous substances that they may use during the course of their work. Within health care, these can range from potentially infected body fluids to microbiological agents, chemicals including disinfectants and gases and dusts. The Regulations place a duty on the employer to provide training related to specific hazards that may be encountered while employed, when new employees begin their jobs or on exposure to new or increased risks. Training should be periodically repeated to refresh knowledge and take place during normal working hours to ensure easy access by the employee to the training being given. The reinforcement of knowledge and training is a feature of health and safety legislation designed to reduce the chances of careless practices developing and thus reduce the risks to the individual worker.

Food-handling

Food and nutrition, essential to life and good health, play a large part in the social life of the human species, and media attention is frequently given to food topics. New strains of bacteria are emerging, and the identification of others hitherto thought to be harmless but which carry a risk to some groups of clients has raised public awareness of the nature and quality of the food we eat in order to live. In Scotland, an outbreak of food poisoning caused by Escherichia coli 0157 resulted in the deaths of a number of people and was given wide publicity. Pregnant women are routinely advised to avoid eating soft cheeses and pâté in order to avoid listeria poisoning, which will cause little harm to the woman but can affect the fetus.

Previous legislation to ensure that food was wholesome and safe was covered by a number of Acts of Parliament affecting food safety, changes beginning with the Food Act 1984. Further changes were still required as it was recognised that a more comprehensive framework needed to be developed. The result was the 1990 Food Safety Act covering England and Scotland, separate legislation, for constitutional reasons, being required in Northern Ireland. Subject to the Act are food businesses:

'Business' includes activities which would normally be regarded as non-commercial, including the undertaking of a canteen, club, school, hospital or institution and activities or undertakings carried on by a local or public authority. (Howells *et al.* 1990, p. 12)

Under previous legislation, hospitals were effectively protected by Crown Immunity from prosecution for poor food hygiene as legal measures could not be enforced. Historical tradition is respected in that enforcement of the Act remains in the hands of local authorities, who are, especially given the rise in sales of pre-prepared foods, considered to have the best access to local information. 'Local authority enforcement officers have power to inspect and seize unsafe food (s. 9), to serve improvement notices (s. 10) and to obtain prohibition orders to enforce food hygiene regulations (s. 11)' (Howells *et al.* 1990, p. 4). Statistical evidence shows that the number of cases of food contamination continues to rise nationally. Legislation is proposed leading to the development of a new Food Standards Agency, which is expected to take over many of the former functions of the local authority over the next few years. This Food Standards Agency, under the remit of the Minister of Agriculture, is planned to be responsible for food standards, safety and hygiene.

The Food Safety Act 1990 and the Food Safety (General Food Hygiene) Regulations 1995, together with the Food Safety (Temperature Control) Regulations 1995, are the current instruments and are entirely compatible with EC law; as with the Manual Handling of Loads Regulations and COSHH, they feature training as integral to the legislation.

The training of food-handlers is encouraged by the Food Safety Act 1990 and the 1995 Regulations in order that food-handlers may understand the hygiene levels required by the Act and to assist with safe practice.

Thinking point

> Many employers and institutions now encourage their employees to take a course in basic food-handling in line with the Food Safety Act. The certificates in basic food hygiene achieved are often displayed in restaurants and public houses for customers to see, although this is not legally required.
>
> What do you feel might be the advantages of displaying these certificates?

The importance of the supply of safe food to the purchaser is underlined by the penalties imposed by the Act. If found guilty of an offence under the Act, a person may be either fined or imprisoned. In order to prevent the transmission of infection, the 1995 Food Safety Regulations also place responsibility on food-handlers themselves. Food-handlers must ensure that any condition they may have that could transmit through food to another person is notified to the employer, and that they must remain away from work until the condition has cleared. In practice, in order to comply with the Act and to protect their customers, many employers will insist on a general practitioner's medical certificate before permitting a return to work if there is a risk of transmittable illness. Minor cuts on the hands must be covered with plasters, specially designed and coloured bright blue, in order to prevent food contamination. Many employers will also insist that staff who handle food wear gloves at all times when working, as well as protective clothing, for example hats with nets to prevent hair falling into the food.

Do not forget the administrators

An important role in any health care team is played by the administrative staff. The increase in the use of computers for many support tasks, often with the operator sitting in a fixed position, has led to a recognition of the health and safety hazards linked to this type of work. Working at a display screen for long periods can give rise to eye soreness and strain, while sitting in a fixed position may lead to skeletal problems or soft tissue injuries such as repetitive strain injury. As part of the package of health and safety measures dating back to the early 1990s, these risks have been recognised in European law by European Directive 90/270/EEC and in the UK by the Health and Safety (Display Screen Equipment) Regulations 1992. As with other British legislation within the field of health and safety, the Regulations form part of the provisions of the Health and Safety at Work etc. Act 1974, in which responsibility for safe working practices rests with both the employer and the employee.

The Display Screen Regulations apply to people defined as 'users', that is, both employees and any other staff who may be employed by them. Agency staff who are employed in large numbers in health care settings are also partially covered by the Regulations.

In common with other health and safety legislation, the assessment of risk forms the first part of management and the investigation of work station ergonomics. Ergonomics means the 'study of efficiency of persons in their working environment' (Fowler and Fowler 1978, p. 288). The work station includes not only the display screen and computer equipment, but also all other items in the immediate area of the operator, such as a telephone, the chair and any other items forming part of the equipment needed. Employers are also required to ensure that the user of the equipment is able to take breaks away from the equipment, although breaks may take the form of a change of activity. Short frequent breaks from working at the display screen, as opposed to longer periods, are recommended.

Corrective equipment also must be supplied if required. This might well include the provision and use of wrist supports, antiglare screens and other equipment designed to reduce the risk of health problems.

In order to forestall any ophthalmic problems, a recognised complication of work at display screens, the employer is required to provide eyesight tests for employees, although not for agency workers, and may be obliged to provide spectacles for the employee if it can be shown that they are necessary.

Despite these highly specific measures, it must be remembered that administrators are equally subject to health and safety legislation, as will be any other employee. For example, the Manual Handling Regulations 1992 are as applicable to a person lifting photocopy paper or stores as they are to the moving and handling of dependent patients.

Conclusion

Health and safety are vital to the efficient delivery of quality care by all those involved with clients. The safe delivery of care involves all aspects of nursing and therapy work.

The safe administration of drugs, and the monitoring of good and bad side-effects, is vital in the treatment of many clients. Health care workers need to be aware of the need to report any changes in their clients to a registered professional, who can then assess the effects of the treatment that has been prescribed. The Medicines Act 1968 controls the prescription and sale of the majority of the drugs used in modern health care, from the humble pack of paracetamol purchased on the way home to powerful modern drugs.

The Health and Safety at Work etc. Act 1974 acts as an 'umbrella' for much of the legislation produced in Europe and aims to provide safe working conditions in which all groups of health care workers can work together without risk to their clients. As the Health and Safety at Work etc. Act 1974 acts as an umbrella, it is comparatively easy to add new items, and currently being adopted are the Regulations concerning safe working hours, designed to ensure that all workers take adequate breaks and rest periods.

In health and safety matters, advice for the employee is available for employers from the offices of the Health and Safety Executive based in larger towns throughout England and Scotland. For employees, advice is available either from the Executive's offices or from trade unions for those who are paid-up members. Unions have health and safety representatives and train their representatives in the specific type of risk associated with the industry in which the member is working. Advice is available either from the health and safety representatives, many of whom have taken a formal part in the workplace risk assessment, or through the permanent officers of the union based in a regional or head office.

References and further reading

Bennett B and Howells R (1997) *Occupational Health and Safety Law* (3rd edn). London, M & E Pitman

Department of Health (1989) *The Control of Substances Hazardous to Health: Guidance for the Initial Assessment in Hospitals*. London, HMSO

Downie G, Mackenzie J and Williams A (1995) *Pharmacology and Drug Management for Nurses*. Edinburgh, Churchill Livingstone

Fowler F and Fowler H (1978) *The Oxford Handy Dictionary*. London, Chancellor Press

Health and Safety Executive (1996) *RIDDOR, Everyone's Guide to RIDDOR '95*. London, HSE

Health and Safety Advisory Committee (1992) *Guidance on Manual Handling of Loads in the Health Services*. London, HMSO

House of Commons, Committee on Safety and Health at Work (1972) (Chairman, Lord Robens) Safety and Health at Work, Report of the Committee 1970–1972. London, HMSO

Howells G, Bradgate R and Griffiths M (1990) *Blackstone's Guide to the Food Safety Act 1990*. London, Blackstone Press

Jenkins R (1995) *The Law and the Midwife*. Oxford, Blackwell Scientific

Kitson A, Brown J and McKnight T (1992) *Challenges in Caring: Explorations in Nursing and Ethics*. London, Chapman & Hall

Logan P (1996) Moving and handling: protecting yourself. *Community Nurse*, April: 22–4

Marshall E (1995) *General Principles of Scots Law* (6th edn). Edinburgh, W Green & Son

Montgomery J (1997) *Health Care Law*. Oxford, Oxford University Press

Rogers R, Salvage J and Cowell R (1999) *Nurses at Risk: A Guide to Health and Safety at Work*. Basingstoke, Macmillan

Royal College of Nursing (1996) *Hazards of Nursing: Personal Injuries at Work*. London, RCN

Royal Pharmaceutical Society of Great Britain (1994) *The Administration and Control of Medicines in Residential and Children's Homes*. London, RPSGB

Smith I, Goddard C and Randall N (1993) *Health and Safety: The New Legal Framework*. London, Butterworth

Stranks J (1994) *Human Factors and Safety*. London, Pitman

Chapter 5 Care in the community

- Background and the concept of care in the community
- Acute care in the community and the primary care team
- The care plan and funding issues
- Continuing care and the key players
- Disability and the physically disabled client
- References and further reading

Background and the concept of care in the community

The NHS as we know it was introduced by Section 6 of the NHS Act 1948, with subsequent statutes supporting the concept of the wholesale provision of health care. The largely discretionary National Assistance Act 1948, on the other hand, was the first significant piece of legislation to direct social services to provide certain services on the basis of their sound judgement. For example, Section 47 of the National Assistance Act 1948 enabled local authorities to remove from their homes, and place into care, those who might be a danger to themselves or others. As provided by the amended Section 27 of that Act:

a local authority may, with the approval of the Secretary of State, and to such an extent as he may direct shall make arrangements for providing: (a) Residential care for persons aged 18 or over who by reason of age, illness, disability or any other circumstances are in need of care and attention which is not otherwise available to them.

Other related legislation includes the Public Health Acts and the Chronically Sick and Disabled Persons Act 1970, which places a legal obligation on agencies to act in the interest of clients falling within the Act.

The Chronically Sick and Disabled Persons Act 1970 marked a move from the discretionary provisions of the National Assistance Act 1948 in that it required local authorities to provide services for disabled people who lived within their area. The rights of disabled people were further consolidated by the Disability Discrimination Act 1995, which supports disabled individuals, while defining new rights in employment and in the acquisition of goods and services as well as enhancing their property law rights.

One of the most important statutes in the history of the NHS was the NHS and Community Care Act 1977, which laid the basis for health care Trusts, both acute hospital-based Trusts and those in the community.

The importance of informal care – that is, the care provided by relatives and friends for disabled or elderly individuals – is recognised by the Carers (Recognition and Services) Act 1995. This statute defines the rights of carers, provided the client is known to the social services, and clarifies the provision for an assessment under Section 1(a) of the NHS and Community Care Act 1990. The Act also asserts the carer's right to an assessment prior to the client's discharge from hospital.

On a practical level, community care should be seen as the sum total of many aspects and facets of provision and care services for clients within a home or community-based institutional setting. Others see it as a 'jigsaw puzzle' and describe it as 'a combination of support services for persons with care needs' (Meredith 1995, p. 17)

Before 1993, earlier legislation stipulated what the health authorities, and similarly local authority social services departments, were empowered to provide by law. NHS health authorities (which are also responsible for general practitioners, dentists and opticians working in the community) provided mainly acute services together with some long-term nursing care for the elderly and in psychiatry. Social services, on the other hand, tended to provide the bulk of any social care, of which the home help service is an example.

The effect of the NHS and Community Care Act 1990 has been to shift the balance from the acute hospital sector to the community. The professionals involved in this process are not only NHS health care professionals, but also social workers, charity-funded workers (for example, Macmillan nurses who work with the terminally ill) and private concerns, who play an important part in looking after the elderly requiring long-term care.

The role of the purchasers – the health authorities – is to buy services on behalf of the clients from the providers, having been allocated proportionate funding from the DoH. Other purchasers of health care are family health practitioner authorities and fundholding general practitioners. In particular, fundholding general practitioners may purchase a range of services covering the multidisciplinary approach. The fundholders are seen as the cornerstone of development in the NHS, with the eventual development of primary care groups and primary health care Trusts.

The term 'primary care' is now used for the provision of all types of health care within the community, involving professionals from many disciplines. Primary care includes not only the provision of acute and long-term care, but also measures to prevent ill-health and to maintain the health of the local community.

Acute care in the community and the primary care team

The publication of the DoH's White Paper *The New NHS: Modern, Dependable* (Department of Health 1997) has reinforced the trend towards the provision of more acute care within the community sector, a trend that is mirrored in Scotland by the White Paper entitled *Designed to Care: Renewing the National Health Service in Scotland* (Scottish Office 1997). A further contributory factor in the provision of acute services in the community has been the growth in the rate of day surgery and treatment over the past decade. The provision of day surgery is seen partly as a response to a call for the reduction of surgical waiting lists and partly as the result of improved methods of anaesthesia and advances in surgical technique. However, Sutherland (1996, p. 5) describes how day surgery was undertaken on paediatric cases as early as 1909 in Scotland when the surgeon 'performed minor orthopaedic procedures on these children as day cases and immediately returned them to their mother's arms, allowing them home to recover in familiar surroundings'. The cumulative effect of governmental policies, earlier discharge from hospital and the treatment of both medical and surgical patients as day cases has resulted in the community health care team being increasingly concerned with acute short-term, as well as more traditional long-term, care. This change of focus has resulted in the development of multidisciplinary primary care teams working within the community setting.

> List the health care professionals who work within the community setting.
>
> If you are working in the community, or are about to do so, consider which other professional groups will interlink with the health care workers.
>
> If you are working within a hospital, find out how the link is made with the professionals in the community.

The importance of links being formed by health care professionals within the community is emphasised by the White Papers that state that social services should be represented on NHS Trust boards in order to facilitate greater co-operation between social work and health care in the community. The role and functions of district nurses, health visitors and community midwives are likely to be extended further. 'The Government is particularly keen to extend the recent developments in the roles of nurses working within acute and community services' (Department of Health 1997, p. 46). The importance of forming links with all groups involved is also seen as essential:

GPs and the general practice team need to work closely with community nurse, midwives and therapists to offer comprehensive and appropriate support to their patients. Community pharmacists, dentists and ophthalmic opticians provide essential services, and access to their skills and professional expertise can greatly enhance the effectiveness of the team. (Scottish Office 1997, p. 18)

In order further to extend the remit of primary care, the NHS (Primary Care) Act 1997 allows groups of professionals the chance to provide care for those, among others, 'who are often alienated from traditional service provision' (Gardner 1998, p. 21). Examples of how this is being developed are existing schemes where health visitors and nurses are working as special-ist practitioners with refugees and asylum-seekers, travellers and their families, and young carers. The 1996 Asylum and Immigra-tion Act removed the automatic right to financial and housing support from the state. 'However, all refugees, including asylum seekers, are entitled to hospital treatment and health services through general practitioners, under the same arrangements as other residents in the UK' (Jobbins 1997, p. 166). Much of the contact with this group and with people from ethnic minorities is being made by health visitors working within a specialist role. Similarly, specialist needs have been identified among traveller families defined by the Caravan Sites Act 1968 as 'Persons of nomadic habit of life whatever their race or origin' (Anderson 1997, p. 148). The travelling families reported that their major points of contact with health service personnel were through midwives visiting pregnant women and through health visitors. Despite this, poor levels of health care uptake have been identi-fied, and a health visitor has been appointed to act as a specialist practitioner to meet the needs of the travelling families. The plight of child carers is a concern for all members of the multi-professional team who work with children, including teaching staff as well as health care professionals. Support for young children who act as carers to disabled adults may be given by youth workers, but school nurses, health visitors and district nurses may all play a part in reducing the stress of this particular group of children, who have a right to services under the Carers (Recognition and Services) Act 1995.

Prescribing by nurses from a limited list is now a reality in some parts of the country and is likely to expand. The Medicinal Products: Prescription by Nurses Act 1992 has been piloted, and a list of substances that may be prescribed is given in the *British National Formulary*. In one pilot reported by Smith (1996, p. 8), 12 nurses working in rural Scotland all received in-service training in order that they might prescribe from the nurses' limited list. The greater contact that the nurses have with the clients in the area has resulted in a potentially more efficient nursing service, although it is noted that the scheme relies heavily on a close working relation-ship between the nurse and the general practitioner.

The development of rapid response teams and 'hospital at home' care also demonstrates how professionals, health care workers and social workers in the primary health care sector may collaborate. In these schemes, clients who fall acutely ill at home remain there supported by the necessary agencies until recovery occurs or other long-term arrangements can be made. Support may include the administration of drugs by the intravenous route, a move that entails the further training of registered nurses working in the community as this route was formerly used exclusively within the hospital sector. Drug administration by this route is an example of how the move from a more long-term picture of care has altered towards acute care delivery within the community. In order to ensure that adequate blood levels of the prescribed drug are maintained, administration needs to conform to a strict timetable. This requires a high degree of time-planning by nurses, who need to take into account considerations such as these when planning their visits to clients. This position may be slightly ameliorated in some areas where hospital at home care is delivered by teams specifically dedicated to the care of the acutely ill in the community. Informal carers who are family members or friends are sometimes involved in this process and are often taught care procedures, including some advanced skills, in order to give the client the best possible support.

The increasing focus on primary health care, that is, care within the community, gives rise to ethical questions of autonomy on the part of the client and the practitioner. The client is being treated within his own home, reinforcing his or her right to autonomy. 'Autonomous people make their own unhampered decisions about how they are going to live' (Bird and White 1995, p. 118), and imposing care is far more difficult than in a hospital, when a client may well feel more defenceless. Care will need to be negotiated by the professionals with the client and carer in order to achieve a successful outcome. In the primary care setting, care delivery is far more client centred, and, in order to achieve this, health care professionals and workers need to have well-developed communication networks in which the client is fully involved. In many cases, this will mean that the care records are held by the clients or their carers, who are also encouraged to enter records. However, this does not absolve the health care team from making a full and clear record of all care delivered. For health care workers, in the occurrence of an investigation, if something is not recorded, it will be treated as not having happened at all as there will be no proof that the action took place. It is difficult to speculate at present how the use of increasingly sophisticated technology, such as laptop computers, for record-keeping will develop within primary care. The government White Papers for both England and Scotland highlight the need to utilise information technology to make best use of resources and the close link that resource has with record-keeping within primary care in the client's own home. For example, a patient's record may include the dressings used, which then have to be replenished. The use of a laptop computer with a modem can allow a health care professional to link with a central site in order to reduce the number of official trips that have to be made and consequently increase the time that can be spent with clients. In an urban area, this may be a comparatively simple matter, whereas in rural areas, travel to and from an official base can be time consuming. However, resource considerations would not permit each client to have a laptop computer in the home, which immediately brings into question the amount of information that could then be held by the client. Consideration also needs to be given to the provisions of the Data Protection Act 1984 and the position of confidential information held in electronic form.

Representation of the client's interests can be supported by the community health councils (CHCs). CHCs were set up during the mid-1970s to promote and support patient-centred care, and represent patients both in the hospital and in the community. In England and Wales, there are about 200 CHCs at present, with similar organisations in Scotland and Northern Ireland. In addition to representing patients' interests, the CHC visits hospital and community homes to ensure that adequate standards of care are being met. Patient interests may also be represented through the Patient's Association as well as through community and hospital Trust routes.

The care plan and funding issues

The White Paper *Caring for People in the Next Decade and Beyond* (Department of Health 1989), published by the Conservative government, saw the role of the NHS, including community-based care, as one of aiming to improve health, with targets to achieve, and to improve systems of accountability. The Labour government, elected in 1997, has a stated policy in its two White Papers of continuing this philosophy. Subject to Section 46 of the NHS and Community Care Act 1990, the social service departments of local authorities have a statutory duty to consult other agencies, principally health authorities, when drawing up their budgetary allocation. This forms the basis of the social service community care plan showing the allocation of resources in the short term and giving a 5-year financial plan for the delivery of social care. This overall view is reflected in the process of formulating an individual care plan in which clients must be consulted and their needs given maximum consideration. In both scenarios, the competing demands of all groups must be balanced (Teasdale 1992, pp. 1 and 3). It is clear that the limited resources argument has been used successfully in the courts to justify the local authority or health authority's inability to meet those demands (Clements 1997, p. 24).

For the client who needs a residential or nursing home placement, the starting point for the process is a financial assessment, which is currently means tested. At the present time, the first £10 000 of capital is ignored, with a contribution being required from the client on a rising scale until a ceiling of £16 000 is reached, after which the client is expected to meet all or part of the cost of care. Any periodic increase in the contribution is linked to inflation. These financial considerations have led to difficulty in the discharge of dependent, mostly elderly, clients from hospital and into the community, and to the phrase 'bed-blockers' being used to describe the plight of clients who require nursing rather than hospital care but lack the funds to pay for it. The consequence is that they must remain in hospital occupying an acute bed until the social services budget permits their discharge into residential care. One promising possibility is the development of intermediate care facilities for the elderly patient. In intermediate care, clients who have received acute care but are not yet ready for discharge, still requiring some level of nursing and rehabilitation, are transferred to a less acute setting. Once ready, they can then either return home or move to a more sheltered setting suitable for their needs.

For the client who is able to be discharged home, charges are also made for social services, a common example being that of home carers, formerly the 'home help' service. Charges for these services vary from authority to authority. Clients who are able to afford it may also purchase their own services from privately run agencies.

Thinking point

> Ronald is a 78-year-old widower who has no family. Ronald is not happy with his new home carer, who, he says, spends most of her time social-ising with him and sometimes fails to turn up.
>
> He has the resources to pay for private home care but is not prepared to do so as a matter of principle.
>
> Should he complain to social services, who he knows are stretched, or should he employ a private carer?

Statistical evidence shows that the population of the UK has increased since the inception of the NHS in 1948 and that this increase is particularly marked in relation to the proportion of elderly people in the population. As people now live longer, they will tend to require greater health care services. Because of pressure from rising costs, it is therefore more viable for the long-term care of the elderly to be provided by the private sector and a clear distinction to be made between the client's assessed needs for nursing and for personal care, as suggested by the NHS and Community Care Act 1990. The stark choice facing the depen-dent client and relatives is basically one of the following:

- Care in the home, care being delivered by NHS health care professionals and some private input
- Residential care provided either by the private sector or, for the poorest, the local authority
- Nursing home care, principally provided by the private sector.

A further option is that of care in the home, this being deliv-ered by a spouse or a close family relative, and in some cases friends and neighbours, collectively known as informal – that is, unpaid – carers. It is such individuals that the Carers (Recogni-tion and Services) Act 1995 is aimed at assisting. The Act gives the right to the carer to be assessed by social services alongside assessment of the client. A recent survey by the Carers National Association showed that fewer than half of the 70 per cent responding said that social services had not told them of their rights, for example to an increase in attendance allowance (George 1997, p. 26). The receipt of attendance allowance would permit informal carers to purchase some services in order to allow them some relief in their caring role.

Thinking point

> Think of two of the clients for whom you care.
>
> Who are the unpaid carers for these clients, and what is their relationship to the client?
>
> Talk to one of the carers about the care they give to the client.

Although there is little or no long-term care being provided by acute health care Trusts, both acute and community Trusts in many areas provide day hospital facilities in order to deliver specialist assessment together with appropriate referral to services required, as well as some treatment. This form of day care may be led by either general practitioners or consultant medical practitioners within an acute hospital Trust.

Continuing care and the key players

The effect of changing health care policy has seen a mushrooming of residential homes, particularly for elderly clients, and the evolution of a huge employment sector for health care workers. Many of these residential homes have dedicated units for, or will accept, younger clients who have long-term nursing needs. There is also a significant health care sector, principally charitably funded, catering for the needs of chronically ill and disabled clients with specific conditions. Those who have long-term care needs are usually recognised for the first time following an acute hospital admission, when assessment is made and a decision – in partnership with the client – made on whether residential placement is more suitable than home care. A nursing needs assessment is also carried out to determine whether a nursing home or 'rest home' will be most appropriate to meet clients' needs. This assessment will include the consideration of such factors as how independently self-caring they may be, risk assessment for falls and the effects of medication.

In the case of the semi-independent elderly person, sheltered accommodation may be suitable, with a warden on call in case of emergencies and home carer (formerly home help) support. This gives the elderly client relative independence as well as the ability to continue to live in the community without going into full-time residential care. Sheltered accommodation is provided both by the local authority, who will require a financial needs assessment, and by the private sector. An increasing quantity of sheltered accommodation is now being provided by housing associations, who are taking the place of the local authorities within the sector. In many cases, the residents in local authority accommodation are former tenants of either the authority or private landlords, having been rehoused in order to free the property they were formerly occupying. Private sector occupiers of sheltered accommodation have, on the other hand, generally sold their own property in order to purchase a purpose-built flat, with the added security of alarm systems for use in an emergency and a warden on call.

For the client who requires a greater degree of care, either residential or nursing home care may be considered. Residential 'rest homes' provide purely for personal services such as safety, food and a degree of supervision and are not required to be managed by a qualified health professional. Nursing homes are required, by the conditions of their local authority licence, to have a registered nurse in charge at all times, aided by care assistants.

There is a legal requirement under the Registered Homes Act 1984 for both residential and nursing homes to be registered with the local authority, be they owned and managed by social services or the private sector. Prior to 1993, residential homes in which no more than four clients were living did not need to be registered, but this was altered by the Registered Homes (Amendment) Act 1991, and now even small homes must be registered with, and open to inspection by, the local authority. Registration with the local authority social services department will state how many residents may live within the home and who is the named manager of the home. The manager and owner are often one and the same, but in cases where the manager is employed by the owner, both must be named on the certificate. Nursing or other care required by a resident in the home is delivered by the primary care team in a fashion similar to that given in the client's own home.

Clients who require a higher level of nursing care as opposed to personal services may need placement in a nursing home. A nursing home is defined by Section 21 of the Registered Homes Act 1984 as one that has 'premises used, or intended to be used, for the reception of, and the provision of nursing for, persons suffering from any sickness, injury or infirmity'. This wide definition is further qualified to cover maternity homes as well as premises in which surgical procedures are carried out. A registered doctor, nurse or midwife must be in charge at all times, the premises must be safe and suitable for the purpose, and the number of clients resident at any one time must not exceed the stated total.

The majority of nursing homes are within the private sector, care being funded either by the client or by social services. Occasionally, as in the case of the hospices, some funding may be via a grant from the health authority. Charitable funding may also play a part in the care of the physically ill or disabled adult within the community. The placement of a client who requires public funding in a nursing home sometimes produces a bottleneck effect as funding needs to be found from social services sources. This bottleneck effect may result in the client having to stay in hospital for some considerable period until both funding and a bed in a suitable nursing home can be found. Registration of a nursing home takes place under Part 2 of the Registered Homes Act 1984, which also makes provision for homes to be dual registered both as a nursing and a residential home in order to provide a continuing service for their residents. The death of clients resident in a nursing home must be reported to the local authority as well as being subject to other statutory notification procedures. Nursing homes are liable to inspection under the 1984 Act, and registration may be removed, with consequent loss of income, if the home is found to be deficient. Action against a nursing home may be taken by the client through the civil route, or by the police if criminal charges are likely.

One type of nursing home that is given widespread public support is the hospice. The philosophy of hospice care was developed in London during 1967 by Cicely Saunders and has spread throughout the country. The hospice movement specialises in the care and support of clients with life-shortening disease, and, although attention has been focused on the care of the cancer victim, hospices also care for those with a variety of other disease conditions. Hospices are registered as nursing homes under the provisions of the Registered Homes Act 1984, and the staff, of all professions, working within the area have expert knowledge in the field of palliative care. Clients are accepted for hospice care on the basis of clinical need rather than the ability to pay.

Funding for a hospice comes from a variety of sources, including health and local authority grants, voluntary contributions and community fundraising efforts. The clients in the hospice are admitted according to need and make a financial contribution only if they are able. A wide variety of health care professionals and workers, together with volunteer staff, care for the clients until death. A recent development has seen the extension of hospice care to the client at home, hospice staff, staff from the Macmillan nursing service and Trust employees working together in order to deliver care within the community.

Hospice care has, in the past, principally focused on the palliative care of cancer patients. The increasing number of AIDS patients during the 1980s has been influential in changing this picture, as a largely young, articulate group of clients demanded high-quality care and symptomatic treatment outside an institutional setting. This shift has seen the adoption of a hospice model of care for other groups, such as those with terminal neuromuscular disorders, for example motor neurone disease.

Thinking point

> What is the name of your local hospice?
>
> Have you seen or heard of any fundraising efforts being made for the hospice?
>
> If possible, establish what conditions are cared for in the hospice.

Disability and the physically disabled client

As the focus of care has shifted towards the care of the physically disabled client in the community as opposed to hospital-based care, it is increasingly important for disabled people, their carers and health care professionals to be aware of the services that are available to the clients.

The 1948 National Assistance Act, one of the major pieces of legislation passed at the end of the 1939–45 war, was aimed at relieving some of Beveridge's categories of want and squalor in relation to the disabled. The Act required local authorities to consider the welfare of adults who were disabled by means of illness or injury and to make known to disabled people the services that the local authority could provide for them. The Act also required the local authority to keep a register of the disabled people known to them, although the later Chronically Sick and Disabled Person's Act 1970 dispenses with formal registration if the client requests it. The 1970 Act requires local authorities to have a knowledge of the number of disabled people resident in the area, to plan for their needs and to publicise services for the disabled. The provisions of the Chronically Sick and Disabled Persons Act 1970 therefore closely resemble those of the later NHS and Community Care Act 1990, which places a similar duty on local authorities to plan and make provision for clients who will require personal care within the community.

The assessment by the local authority of the disabled individual is covered by the Disabled Persons (Services) Act 1986, which closed a gap in the Chronically Sick and Disabled Persons Act by providing for assessment of the client. However, as Montgomery observes:

One key difference between community care services provided by local authorities and those under the NHS is that the former are not free of charge. Local authorities may recover as much of the cost of providing or securing the services as it is reasonably practical for a client to pay. (1997, p. 60)

This may bring with it problems for disabled people, who will be required to pay for some or all of the local authority provision. For many, the answer will be in social security benefits, some of which – attendance allowance being an example – are designed to pay for the purchase of care. Other benefits are means tested, and in the case of a married couple where one partner is in work and supporting a disabled person, his or her income may well disqualify the household from the payment of benefits. Health care professionals who work with disabled people should be aware of to whom to refer them for help and advise on obtaining any benefit that is due to them. The voluntary sector and charitable organisations often offer a great deal of assistance in this situation.

The rights of the carers of disabled people were recognised by the 1995 Carers (Recognition and Services) Act. This Act gives carers the right to be assessed by social services for the provision of assistance in their caring role. However, the disabled person must have been the subject of an assessment by social services prior to recognition of the carer's needs.

The right of disabled people to be part of society as a whole is recognised by the Disability Discrimination Act 1995. The statute has been criticised as it does not provide for a commission to which aggrieved clients may apply in the same way as occurs for other anti-discrimination legislation. Two advisory bodies are set up under the Act to advise the government on disability issues: the National Disability Council, which covers England, Wales and Scotland, and the Northern Ireland Disability Council. The Act does, however, raise awareness and sets out the rights of the disabled person to access, employment and education, and in the buying and selling of property.

References and further reading

Anderson E (1997) Health concerns and needs of traveller families. *Health Visitor* **70**(4): 148–50.

Audit Commission (1994) *Taking Stock, Progress with Community Care No. 2*. London, HMSO

Audit Commission (1996) *Fundholding Facts*. London, HMSO

Bird A and White J (1995) An ethical perspective – patient autonomy. In Tingle J and Cribb A (eds) *Nursing Law and Ethics*. Oxford, Blackwell Scientific, pp. 118–29

Clements L (1997) Rule of Law. *Community Care* **166**: 24–5

Davidson D and Hunter S (1994) *Community Care in Practice*. London, Batsford

Department of Health (1989) *Caring for People in the Next Decade and Beyond*. London, HMSO

Department of Health (1994) *Code of Practice. Mental Health Act 1983*. London, HMSO

Department of Health (1996) *Health Committee 3rd Report (1995–1996). Long Term Care: Future Provision and Funding*, Vol. 1. London, HMSO

Department of Health (1997) *The New NHS: Modern, Dependable*. London, HMSO

Dimond B (1997) *Legal Aspects of Care in the Community*. Basingstoke, Macmillan

Fruin T (1995) *Finding and Funding: Residential Care for the Elderly.* London, Kogan Page

Gardner L (1998) Leading primary care: time for action. *Health Visitor* **71**(1): 21–2

George M (1996) Figure it out. *Community Care* 1–7 August: 2–3

George M (1997) Into the unknown. *Community Care* **1176**: 26–7

Jobbins D (1997) Shelter from the storm. *Health Visitor* **20**(4): 166

Leff J (1997) *Care in the Community: Illusion or Reality.* Institute of Psychiatry. Chichester, John Wiley & Sons

Independent Health Care Association (1995) *An Independent Review of the NHS and Community Care Act, two Years on.* London, Independent Health Care Association

Ineichen B (1992) Managing residential care. *Nursing the Elderly* May/June: 29–30

Jones R (1993) *Registered Homes Manual.* London, Sweet & Maxwell

Meredith B (1995) *The Community Care Handbook* (2nd edn). London, Ace Books

Montgomery J (1997) *Health Care Law.* Oxford, Oxford University Press

Department of Health, Social Services Inspectorate (1996) *Carers (Recognition and Services) Act 1995 Practice Guide.* London. Department of Health/HMSO

Royal College of Psychiatrists of London (1994) *Ensuring Equity and Quality: Case for the Elderly People.* London, Royal College of Psychiatry.

Scottish Office (1997) *Designed to Care: Renewing the National Health Service in Scotland.* Edinburgh, Stationery Office

Skelt A (1993) *Disabilities: Caring for People with Disability in the Community.* London, Pitman

Smith K (1996) Prescriptions in a different hand. *Community Nurse* **2**(7): 8

Sutherland E (1996) *Day Surgery: A Handbook for Nurses.* London, Baillière Tindall/RCN

Teasdale K (1992) *Managing Changes in Health Care* London, Wolfe Publishing

Tierney A and Closs J (1993) Discharge planning for elderly patients. *Nursing Standard* **7**(52): 32

Tomlinson D and Carver J (1996) *Asylum in the Community.* London, Routledge

Tunnicliffe H, Coyle G and More W (1993) *ABC of Community Care.* Birmingham, Pepar

Chapter 6 The child – before and after birth

Introduction

This chapter concentrates on the legal framework surrounding children, relevant ethical issues also being highlighted where necessary. Generally speaking, the term 'child' is used to describe any living being from the time of confinement and birth to below the compulsory school leaving age, that is 16 years or less. The term 'young person' is generally used for those between 16 and the age of legal majority at 18. However, in practice, children develop mentally and physically at wildly different rates, and children between 10 and 14 years of age may be considered as older children, those aged over 14 being viewed as young adults. This brings a peculiar dilemma to the legal approach to children – when is a child not a child?

Family law, or more specifically child law, is part of private law affecting the child. Public law, on the other hand, affects the child indirectly by regulating local authorities in their relationship

95

to the child and other agencies, as well as in the effect of criminal law on the child who commits crime or is a victim of crime.

The first part of the chapter concentrates on the unborn child and is also concerned with another legal and ethical matter, that of the termination of unwanted pregnancy.

As technology advances, the fetus is increasingly being considered as an 'unborn child', and the use of this terminology has become accepted by many. It has been adopted here in recognition of the fact that many contemporary legal and ethical issues surrounding pregnancy and childbirth are centred on the development of a fetus into a child. Not many years ago, *in vitro* fertilisation – test tube babies – was beyond contemporary scientific ability; the use of donor eggs or sperm to create a child was a risky undertaking. Now these procedures have become possible to the extent that many feel that they can claim a right to free treatment for infertility.

Closely linked to issues surrounding the unborn child is the legal definition of biological parenthood. Courts in the USA have recently had to decide who was the legal parent in a complex case in which a couple unable to have children involved sperm and egg donors, the resulting fetus being carried by a surrogate mother. The couple who commissioned the child then divorced, leaving the courts to decide who was responsible for the child's upkeep as she had not been adopted at birth by the couple. The decision was that, as the couple had commissioned the child, expecting to act as parents and responsible for her until adulthood, this wish would stand and the child would be treated as their natural offspring.

The second part of this chapter is devoted to consideration of the child after birth and until the attainment of adult status. Legal and ethical matters concerning the child at home are discussed, together with alternative arrangements that may become necessary as a result of family disruption. Child protection is an important matter for all health care professionals, and one in which the multidisciplinary team may be joined by police officers and others who are concerned with the prevention of child abuse.

The child in hospital, especially the issue of who may give consent to treatment, is considered in the final part of the chapter, along with the child at school and topics related to child employment.

Biological origins

Biologically speaking, living beings emanate directly from their mother. There is no presumption at law that the father is indeed the biological father unless he is married to the mother, and that assumption is, of course, rebuttable, evidence to the contrary being available on a balance of probabilities.

While the unborn child is *in utero* – in the womb – it does not have its own independent existence but total dependence on the mother. However, the mother does not have exclusive rights to the life of the unborn child, and the state may intervene when it feels that the child's rights are in danger of violation. The relationship between the child, its parents and the state is best seen as a tripartite one (Hoggett 1994). The basis of respect for human life, from its very existence, may be based on the United Nations (UN) Declaration (1948) that 'All human beings are born free and equal in dignity and rights'. Adhering to this and other UN declarations, such as the UN Convention on the Rights of the Child 1991, the courts have to adjudicate on behalf of the state where there is dispute over parental responsibility or where the rights of the unborn child are in danger of being overridden (Mason 1998, p. 174).

Parental rights versus children's rights

When a child is in the womb, there is a prima facie – assumed – right of the woman to have a termination under certain provisions of the Abortion Act 1967. The Human Fertilisation and Embryology Act 1990 Section 27(i) states that a pregnant woman who is 'carrying a child or has carried a child as a result of placing in her an embryo or sperm and egg and no other woman is to be treated as the mother of the child', giving the woman the ultimate choice in the matter. However, if fetal rights are abused by a mother who, for example, takes drugs, the courts have been known to section the woman under the Mental Health Acts (England and Scotland) and go as far as ordering a caesarean operation to save the life of the child (McHale *et al.* 1997, p. 942). However, these aspects of law are controversial, create wide discussion in the media and are the subject of much professional debate.

Disputes regarding parental rights have arisen in cases of surrogacy when a mother accepts another's fertilised egg or is fertilised by sperm from a donor. The law on this issue is clear, and the Surrogacy Act 1985 Section 1A clearly places surrogacy agreements outside the law. Although they are not illegal, none of the parties involved can seek a legal redress concerning the arrangement. The legal father is presumed to be the genetic father who is married to the woman, as outlined by Section 26 of the Family Law Reform Act 1969. While the position of the married father is clear, that of the unmarried father is less so. In a paternity claim, a blood test can only establish that the man is not the father of the child; it cannot be used as conclusive proof of paternity, which can be better established by DNA testing.

Until the late 1920s, the traditional role of the father in common law had been one of paternalism – where the father knew what was best for his child and 'regardless of his behaviour or character had an absolute right to entire and untrammelled control over his children until they reached maturity' (Stone 1995, p. 170). The High Court can use its jurisdiction to overturn this traditional view by applying the 'paramountcy principle' to act always in the child's best interest, a view promoted by the philosophy of the Children Act 1989 in England and the Children (Scotland) Act 1995. If necessary, it is possible for the Court to make the unborn child a ward of court and appoint a guardian *ad litem* – normally a social worker – to assume parental responsibility on behalf of the state.

The beginning of life and assisted conception

Human life, in common with most forms of life, begins with the process of reproduction. There is an ongoing debate and dispute over exactly when life begins, this issue being closely examined by both sides in the abortion debate. While there are those who argue that life begins at conception, others would say that life should be valued in stages and that, since the child is incapable of independent existence, it cannot be said to be a person. The role of the law in this situation is to clarify the parameters within which human life is said to exist, while the advance of medical science now makes it possible for ever earlier births to be supported by technological means.

A biologist would assert that every living cell is alive because it is formed by distinguishing characteristics arising from chromosomes. In the human, 46 chromosomes are inherited from the parents at fertilisation, 23 from each parent. Fertilisation is defined as 'the fusion of the nuclei of male and female gametes to form a zygote from which a new individual can develop' (McClean and Jones 1990, p. 100), a gamete being a sex cell containing only 23 chromoses. The zygote, which is the most basic form of advanced life, adheres to the uterus within 4–7 days, as the cells multiply and develop, the cluster of cells is called an embryo until 2 months after fertilisation, then it is described as a fetus until birth.

If the natural method of reproduction fails, it is now possible to employ assisted reproductive techniques. The Human Fertilisation and Embryology Act 1990, together with the revised Human Fertilisation and Embryology Code of Practice 1995, regulates the whole area of assisted reproduction. For a couple who require assisted conception, the process is sometimes laden with frustration: it is estimated that only 40 per cent of couples achieve a successful pregnancy (Donaldson and Donaldson 1993, p. 295). In addition, the cost of treatment to the NHS has resulted in much of the speciality being delivered privately, that is, on a fee-paying basis. Many would argue that infertility is not strictly an illness and that public money should not therefore be allocated to treatment. Hospitals and private clinics that provide assisted conception are licensed by the Human Fertility and Embryology Authority, created by Section 5 of the Human Fertilisation and Embryology Act 1990 and by the Human Fertility and Embryology (Statutory Storage Period) Regulations (SI 1540). Confidentiality of treatment is assured by the Human Fertility and Embryology (Disclosure of Information) Act 1992.

One of the most common ways of artificial insemination is artificial insemination by donor (AID), also known as donor insemination (DI), which is used in the case of male impotence or sterility. The technique is far from new: Cuisine (1990, p. 12) quotes the 1795 case of a London merchant who, suffering from hypospadias, successfully used a syringe to inseminate his wife. The process sometimes involves artificial insemination using frozen sperm from either the woman's husband or a donor. The donor must give permission and consent for the use of his sperm. The practical ethical difficulties of this have been highlighted by the case of Diane Blood, who wished to use sperm extracted from her husband prior to his early death. The husband was unable to give consent because of his illness, although the couple's wish to start a family was known to their relatives. On appeal, the European Court held that Articles contained within the EC treaty applied and could be used to give her the right to have treatment utilising the frozen sperm.

Another, now familiar, method used to assist reproduction – *in vitro* fertilisation – was pioneered as early as 1978 in the UK. A course of hormones is given to the woman in order to stimulate ovulation. The resulting ova are examined microscopically to ensure that they are healthy, are fertilised artificially and are then implanted in the woman's uterus. A donated ovum may be used if a woman is infertile in a process known as gamete interfallopian transfer (GIFT), being mixed with the partner's or donor's sperm and then implanted into the uterus.

Despite the guidance given by law, the whole area of assisted conception – sometimes described as reproductive technology – brings out a huge area of ethical and moral argument. Although some treatments have been known for many years, others are developing rapidly in modern life. There are no real cultural directions on which to base ethical thinking in the area, and the added debate over whether treatment should be available through the NHS or largely privately adds a further dimension to the problem. Nor can earlier generations be referred to guide thinking. Downie and Calman (1994, p. 187) point out that 'There can be no traditional advice on this since it is only recently that the technology has existed, and indeed it is developing every year'. In a situation such as this, the court system may be used to decide the issues using known legal parameters to guide its decisions. Many of these decisions will fall under the philosophical category of utilitarianism in that the action will be right if the greatest good is done in benefiting those affected. Present discussion in the UK is assisted by the report of the Warnock Committee (Department of Health and Social Services 1984), covering wide-ranging topics related to human infertility and its treatment. However, advances in medical technology have in some areas outstripped the report, and further official discussion is likely to take place in order to give advice to health care professionals.

> Should childless couples have the right to assisted conception on the NHS, that is, using public funds?
>
> Should the treatment for infertility be age limited, or should certain circumstances be taken into account when treatment is given? Circumstances could include life history and expectation, financial status and recovery from illness, together with any other factors that you might like to consider.

Research and surrogacy

The whole area of research into embryology and the transplantation or use of fetal cell tissue is again one beset with legal and ethical debate. In addition, it is now possible to operate on a fetus in the womb. The treatment of a fetus *in utero* may cause divided ethical loyalties as the health care team are treating both the pregnant woman and her fetus. As discussed by Beauchamp and Childress (1994, p. 432):

Maternal–fetal relations have recently become more complex and open to conflicts because of the diagnosis and treatment of some maladies in utero – for example, treatment of hydrocephalus through intra-uterine surgery.

Added to this is the possibility of reproducing mammalian life by cloning. In this evolving area, each case must be debated and decided on its merits until sufficient evidence is amassed to provide material for a legal framework.

Surrogacy, sometimes called 'womb-leasing' in the popular press, involves private arrangements to carry a pregnancy that is the result of conception using gametes or a zygote implanted into the surrogate woman. In the UK, such agreements are not enforceable by law and may become a criminal agreement if they infringe adoption legislation under the Adoption Act 1976. Any payments for surrogacy are illegal, although expenses may be payable. Surrogacy arrangements are governed not only by the Adoption Act 1976, but also by the Surrogacy Arrangements Act

1985, and since 1995, a couple may apply for a parental order providing that at least one of them has donated gametes.

Abortion

Abortion has a number of meanings but for the purposes of this chapter can be defined as 'The emptying of the pregnant uterus before the end of the 24th week' (Weller 1997, p. 2). Since April 1968, the Abortion Act 1967 (as amended by the Human Fertilisation and Embryology Act 1990) has allowed abortions up to 24 weeks on the following grounds:

1. that continuation of the pregnancy would involve a risk to the life of the mother or any existing children of her family
2. if necessary to prevent grave permanent injury to the physical or mental health of the woman
3. if there was a substantial risk to the child that it would be born with physical or mental abnormality as to be seriously handicapped. (Young 1992, p. 58)

The issues raised by abortion are extremely controversial, especially in view of technological advances in the support of pre-term deliveries. Ethical and medical debate is also concerned with the exact time at which the fetus can be considered a live being. Abortion is one of the few instances when health care workers and professionals are allowed to opt out under conscientious objection clauses contained within the Abortion Act. This opt-out clause is enshrined in the UKCC's *Code of Professional Conduct* for nurses, midwives and health visitors, although it must be stressed that opt-out is only permissible when it relates to the abortion process and not the care that the woman will require before or after the procedure.

The child at home

The major piece of legislation in England and Wales concerning children both in the home and in local authority care is the Children Act 1989, while in Scotland it is the Children (Scotland) Act 1995. Both Acts repealed and reformed much of the law then existing in relation to the child and its parents, recognising also that children may be housed and cared for under arrangements other than the traditional situation of a child living with its natural parents in their own home.

Society has, through the ages, agreed that a child or children should be bought up by the parents in a home that they provide. The Children Act 1989, in Section 2, replaces the idea of parental 'rights' with the idea that, in order to perform the role of parents, 'parental responsibility' gives a more appropriate and adaptable approach to both parent and child. Parents may be either married or unmarried. If a couple are married, both mother and father share equal parental responsibility for their legitimate offspring until they reach the age of 18. Separation and divorce do not affect parental responsibility for children under the age of 18, divorcing parents being expected to come to agreement, together with their children, on how parental responsibility is to be shared.

A growing number of couples are choosing to have children without the formal legal contract of marriage, and in this case, the mother has automatic parental responsibility for the children under Section 2 of the Family Law Reform Act 1987. The position of the unmarried father is made clearer by Section 4 of the Children Act 1989, which allows a legal parental responsibility agreement to be drawn up and recorded, or alternatively a court order to be made in respect of parental responsibility for the children of the relationship.

Although many health care workers and professionals are involved in the care of the child, one of the key parts is played by the health visitor: 'The role of the health visitor is to provide a service offering advice and help which families are free to accept or reject as they wish' (Robertson 1991, p. 29). The health authority is under a statutory obligation to make provision for health visiting, but, as Robertson states, the family may accept or reject the services of the health visitor. Normally, however, when a woman has given birth, the midwife will notify the health visiting service, usually through a liaison officer, giving some basic information from which the health visitor can work. Although much of the health visitor's workload is concerned with the health and welfare of young children, including child abuse, health visiting is also concerned with the welfare of the elderly and the handicapped.

A growing number of children, some of very tender years indeed, have been found to be acting as carers for a disabled person, usually a parent, within the home. Smith (1997, p. 137) identifies that 'As many as 50,000 young people in the UK may be carers, looking after a disabled or long-term sick parent or siblings at home.' The Carers (Recognition and Services) Act 1995 emphasises that, when such cases come to the notice of social services, the needs of the child to be a child first and a carer second must be recognised in the provision of services. It should be noted, however, that before this provision can be made, the disabled person in the home must have first been assessed by social services.

The parents are expected to provide a home, in its broadest sense, for their child in order to give shelter, warmth and food as well as the less tangible provisions of emotional security and stability.

Removal of the child from the home without legal authority could result in criminal proceedings being taken against the abductor. Legal decisions concerning the removal of a child from the family home may be particularly difficult during the early stages of divorce proceedings when custody has not been decided, and it may be that the police are unable to take any action for abduction in the absence of an agreement by the parents regarding the place of the child's home. Sections 49–51 of the Children Act 1989 recognise the risk of abduction and give a statutory framework for the necessary action to be taken in order to return the child to its place of legal residence.

If there is a risk of abduction abroad, either responsible parent may request that a passport is issued to a child only with their knowledge. In normal circumstances, the consent of one person with parental responsibility is required before a passport can be issued to a child under the age of 16, or the children may be included on the parent's own passport.

Child protection

Child protection, with its necessary implication of child abuse, is an emotive and difficult subject in which private law and both civil and criminal divisions of public law may be involved. Equally difficult is a definition of the word 'abuse'. Meadow (1997, p. 1) suggests that 'A child is considered to be abused if he or she is treated in a way that is unacceptable in a given culture at a given time.' This poses difficulties for any multicultural – as opposed to multiethnic – society, in which standards of what is, or is not, acceptable may vary widely. Health care workers, both within their professional work and as members of society, may be in a better position than many to recognise possible signs of child abuse by the physical and behavioural manifestations of differing types of abuse.

Physical abuse is possibly the simplest type of abuse to detect. Physical abuse leaves visible signs of injury, such as bruising, thermal injury or fractures, on a child's body. Although these signs may be hidden by clothing, the child's body language indicating pain might give a clue to non-accidental injury, as could crying, grizzling or, even more worryingly, silence and withdrawal. In children who are old enough to speak, the story of how the injury was caused might not agree with the injury that has been detected, or conflicting histories may be given by the child and the parent. Medical advice is unlikely to have been sought in respect of the child's injuries.

Thinking point

> How might a child show signs of pain? Consider both verbal, that is, audible, signs and non-verbal signs, that is, those signs often described as body language.
>
> Children of different ages are likely to show pain in a variety of ways. How might pain be recognised in a very young child and in the older child?

A further category of physical abuse, one so serious that it deserves a classification all of its own, is that of sexual abuse. Sexual abuse may involve any type of sexual behaviour that is performed on a child by an adult, including anal, vaginal or oral penetration. The DoH (1991) defines sexual abuse as:

the involvement of dependent, immature children and adolescents in sexual activity which they do not really comprehend, to which they are unable to give informed consent, which violate the social taboos of family life and which are knowingly not prevented by the carer.

Sexual abuse may be difficult to detect as the child is often reluctant to admit that it has occurred, or he or she might have been bribed by gifts or money not to tell.

Two types of child abuse are closely related to the Children Acts' (England and Scotland) expectation of parental responsibility in that the responsibilities of being a parent in relation to food, psychological security and possibly even shelter are failing, to the detriment of the child's health. Abuse by neglect features a failure to provide suitable food, clothing or housing for the child. The child, as a result of the abuse, shows poor physical and mental growth and frequent ill-health. Emotional abuse ranges from a failure to provide for the psychological needs of the child in respect of love and cognitive development to outright verbal abuse, verbal bullying and disparagement of the child's ability. The suspicion of both neglect and emotional abuse is closely linked to the child's failure to reach accepted physical and psychological developmental milestones or to inappropriate behaviours such as self-mutilation, compulsive stealing or scavenging.

Child protection is an important feature of the Children Acts 1989 and 1995, and requires a multidisciplinary approach with health care professionals working in collaboration for child protection measures to be effective.

Thinking point

How many groups of professionals, from all backgrounds, might come into contact with:

● The pre-school child
● The child at school?

The death in 1973 of Maria Colwell, a child who had suffered the most horrific abuse and whose case was widely publicised at the time, being remembered to this day, highlighted the number of professional groups that come into contact with children. Many of them were aware of the abuse that Maria was suffering, and each group was trying to take some action to alleviate her situation. However, each group was working in isolation, and the resulting enquiry recommended that interagency collaboration and co-ordination were vital in order to reduce the risk of a similar situation occurring again. While the Children Acts are concerned with the protection of children at risk of abuse, the principal guidance for interagency collaboration in England is given by the DoH publication *Working Together under the Children Act: A Guide to Arrangements for Inter-agency Co-operation for the Protection of Children from Abuse* (1991). Area child protection committees (ACPCs) take the lead in this role, all agencies concerned with child protection meeting together. Representatives on the committee are drawn from health care services – both hospital and community, including those caring for physical as well as mental health, and drawn from both nursing and medicine – education, social services and the police. Other important agencies are also represented, the National Society for the Prevention of Cruelty to Children (NSPCC) being particularly prominent. The legal services are also represented, with the courts, the probation service and the Crown Prosecution Service being included in the ACPC. As with any working group, other professionals with particular interest and expertise to offer may be co-opted to serve on either the main committee or a sub-committee. As the ACPC is a large group, sub-committees are formed to meet specific needs identified by the group as a whole. These sub-committees meet more frequently than the full ACPC and are responsible for the day-to-day work of co-ordinating child protection, developing policies and guidelines to assist professionals in dealing with suspected abuse and training staff in the action that should be taken.

An overall body such as the ACPC is unable to deal with individual cases of children who are suspected to be the victims of child abuse, so the policies and guidelines developed by the sub-committees become invaluable to the practitioner working with children. These policies and guidelines will outline the action to be taken when abuse is suspected. Once the likelihood of abuse is recognised, a case conference is the next step. At the case conference, the family and the professionals involved with the child meet to discuss the child and to agree how action should be taken.

In order to provide information on a child's risk to all agencies involved with children, a Child Protection Register is kept. The Register is most usually kept by social services, and professional staff of all disciplines who work with children have access to it on a named basis. The Register will have details of the child and the protection plan developed at the case conference and is reviewed regularly so that progress and the support provided can be assessed. Although the Children Act 1989 is the major statute, some amendment has been introduced by the Family

Law Act 1996, in that a court may rule that a person who is suspected of child abuse within one of the four categories is to be excluded from the child's home while an emergency protection order is in force.

Children and the local authority

The local authority, specifically social services, plays an important part in the care of children whether living in the family home or resident in homes provided by the local authority (children in care). This section is designed to give the reader an overview of the local authority's involvement with the child who lives at home as opposed to the child who is living in the care of the local authority. For children in local authority care, the reader should consult the literature on child care within social services provision.

Part 3 of the Children Act 1989 focuses on the local authority's involvement with the child who lives at home, specified as 'in need' by Section 17 of the Act. The section is wide ranging and covers children in all situations. Children who may require social services help while still living in their home can be summarised as those:

- Who are unlikely to be able to develop normally and in good health without some local authority support
- Whose condition may become even worse without support
- Who are disabled.

Schedule 2 of the Act gives the local authority guidance on how children in need are to be identified, and a register of disabled children is to be kept. The local authority's services are to be publicised, being translated if necessary into minority languages in order to promote access. Assessment of the services that both the child and the family may require is logically the first step once their need has been recognised. The provision of services can then be planned to meet the requirements that have been recognised. The services may range from practical help such as home help, although payment for these may be required, through the psychological assistance of counselling and advice.

The Children Act 1989 is concerned with guardianship of the child both in the private law area of family law and the public law area, in which the local authority is involved. One form of guardianship concerns the appointment, under Section 41 of the Act, of a guardian *ad litem*, a social worker, to represent the child and to safeguard the child's interests during court proceedings. These proceedings may include court orders being made in respect of child protection as well as other occasions when a child's welfare is paramount. The guardian *ad litem* has wide-ranging responsibilities and powers in order to effectively represent the child to the court and when a welfare report is required by the court. The importance of adequate representation of the child is supported by the Family Law Act 1996, under which the child's wishes must be considered during divorce proceedings and when settlement is made, although a guardian *ad litem* may not necessarily be involved in this process.

The appointment of a guardian under Part 1 of the Act, which deals with parenting matters, is the arrangement whereby:

A guardian is an individual who stands in place of a parent with parental responsibility for the child, and may consent, or withhold consent, to adoption. He may be appointed by a parent who has parental responsibility for the child, a guardian of the child or the court. (Harris and Scanlan 1991, p. 7)

Logically, to prevent confusion, the appointment of a guardian to act in the stead of a parent must be made in writing and may be accompanied by a residence order made through the court. An example of when guardianship may be necessary is the case of a terminally ill single or divorced parent who wishes to ensure their children's care after death.

The child in hospital/informed consent

The issue of who gives consent to treatment when a child requires medical treatment or care is one that is fraught with both legal and ethical difficulties. Although very few health care professionals would be willing or able to treat an unco-operative child, it can become necessary for the child, that is, a person under the age of 16, to have treatment. Once the child has attained the age of 16, and in the absence of any known mental illness or handicap, they are assumed to have sufficient understanding to give informed consent to treatment on their own behalf.

For a young child, the issues are comparatively simple: the written consent to treatment is signed by either the parent or the guardian of the child on the basis of his or her informed consent, in which an understanding of potential risks has been reached and outweighed by the benefits of the proposed treatment. In this situation, the guardian is the appointed person who has assumed parental responsibility for the child.

However, the situation becomes more difficult as children get older and are able to express their wishes. One major ethical issue concerns the prescription of contraception to girls under the age of 16 without parental or guardian consent. This issue was bought to public debate by Mrs Victoria Gillick, who argued against DoH advice to doctors that they could lawfully prescribe contraception to a girl under 16 years of age and that parental rights would be breached if the prescription were written without parental consent. Mrs Gillick's objections were made through the courts and reached the House of Lords, who ruled that if a child could achieve sufficient comprehension to understand completely the treatment proposed, with both its benefits and side-effects, the child could give informed consent on his or her own behalf. The House of Lords decision has become known as 'Gillick competence', and doctors may now prescribe for, or treat, children under the age of 16 providing they meet the requirements of understanding.

This calls into question the whole idea of parental rights, as once a child has achieved Gillick competence and until the age of 16, both the parent/guardian and the child may give consent to treatment. Despite this, it needs to be recognised that many children as well as adults may achieve understanding on one matter only to fail to achieve it on another. Thus an assessment of each individual is vital in relation to any proposed treatment.

In Scotland, the Age of Legal Capacity (Scotland) Act 1991 gives guidance to health care professionals. In general, children below the age of 16 may not enter legally binding agreements, although health care provides some exceptions:

A child under 16 may consent to any surgical, medical or dental procedure or treatment where, in the opinion of the medical practitioner attending him or her, the child is capable of understanding the nature and possible consequences of the procedure or treatment. (Fabb and Guthrie 1997, p. 80)

In both England and Scotland, the need for an individual assessment of a child's comprehension and reasoning capability is essential before consent to treatment can be gained, and the child's capacity for refusal of treatment is even more problematical. This aspect of care is given little support by the law, although it requires a greater understanding on the part of the child of the long-term outcome if treatment is refused.

The child at school and at work

Health care professionals who are in contact with children need to be aware of the legislation concerning children's schooling and any employment that children undertake as both of these may have an effect on their health and development. Detailed knowledge is not essential for the delivery of health care but may help the professional in assessing the world in which the child lives as opposed to his or her direct health care needs.

The Children Act 1989 describes parental responsibilities towards the child as including that of education. School-age children must be in full-time education suitable to their needs. The Education Acts of 1980, 1981 and 1988 contain the law on the education of children, those of 1980 and 1988 giving parents preference over school choice and religious practice within school, while the Education Act of 1988 is of particular interest to those who are working with children who have special needs.

As the section on child protection has shown, many professional groups are concerned with the welfare of the child, and some recognition of the law concerning education and child employment is of interest to those whose practice covers children. The importance of education for a child's psychological development and future prospects is acknowledged by Section 36 of the Children Act 1989, which allows for the making of an Education Supervision Order (ESO). The Order requires that a supervisor 'must advise, assist and befriend, and may give directions to, a child and his parents with a view to seeing that the child is properly educated, taking into account the wishes and feelings of both the parents and the child' (Harris and Scanlan 1991, p. 17). Thus the ESO, in line with the philosophy of the Children Act, involves the whole family, together with the education authority, which seeks the Order, to achieve benefit for the child.

The employment of children is a difficult subject. Many children wish to work in order to gain experience, other children may have to work in order to supplement the family income, while others are made to work. In order to protect the interests of children working, there are legally enforceable controls on when children may or may not work. For the purposes of employment, the distinction between children – those of compulsory school age – and young persons aged 16–18 is an important one. Legal restrictions principally refer to the employment of children, the Employment Act of 1989 having removed the limitations on the 16–18 year age group. Statutory controls over younger children are still governed by the Children and Young Persons Act 1933, which rules that children may not be employed if they under 13 years old, during school hours, before 7 a.m., or after 7 p.m. or for more than 2 hours a day, and that they may not lift, carry or move heavy objects that might injure them. Although containing no specific guidance with respect to child employment, health and safety legislation also forms an important legal framework and is as applicable to children as it is to adult employees.

References and further reading

Alderson P (1990) *Choosing for Children: Parents Consent to Surgery.* Oxford, Oxford University Press

Allen N (1992) *Making Sense of the Children Act* (2nd edn). Harlow, Longman

Bainham A and Gretney S (1993) *Children – the Modern Law.* Bristol, Family Law/Jordan Publishing

Beauchamp J and Childress J (1994) *Principles of Biomedical Ethics* (4th edn). Oxford, Oxford University Press

Cuisine D (1990) *The New Reproductive Technique – a Legal Perspective.* Aldershot, Dartmouth

Department of Health (1991) *Working Together under the Children Act: A Guide to Arrangements for Interagency Co-operation for the Protection of Children from Abuse.* London, HMSO

Department of Health and Social Services (1984) Report of the Committee of Inquiry into Human Fertilization and Embryology (the Warnock Report). London, HMSO

Donaldson R and Donaldson L (1993) *Essential Public Health Medicine.* Lancaster, Kluwer Academic

Downie A (1997) The doctor and the teenager – questions of consent. *Family Law* **27**: 499–501

Downie R and Calman K (1994) *Healthy Respect: Ethics in Health Care* (2nd edn). Oxford, Oxford Medical Publications

Eekelaar J and Dingwall R (1990) *The Reform of Child Care Law: A Practical Guide to Children Act 1989*. London, Tavistock/Routledge

Fabb J and Guthrie T (1997) *Social Work Law in Scotland*. London, Butterworth

Fish D (1997) Child abuse – a legal practitioners guide. *Family Law* **27**: 666

Fyfe C (1995) *The Layman's Guide to Scotland's Law*. Edinburgh, Mainstream Publishing

Harris P and Scanlon D (1991) *The Children Act 1989: A Procedural Handbook*. London, Butterworth

Hendrick J (1993) *Child Care Law for Health Professionals*. Oxford, Radcliffe Medical Press

Mason J (1998) Medico-legal aspects of reproduction and parenthood (2nd edn). Aldershot, Dartmouth, pp. 174–6

McHale J, Fox M and Murphy J (1997) *Health Care Law, Text and Materials*. London, Sweet & Maxwell

McClean D & Jones B (1990) *Introduction to Human and Social Biology*. London, Butler & Tanner

Meadow R (1997) *ABC of Child Abuse* (3rd edn). London, BMJ Publishing

Murphy M (1995) *Working Together in Child Protection: An Exploration of the Multidisciplinary Task and System*. Aldershot, Arena

Robertson C (1991) *Health Visiting in Practice* (2nd edn). Edinburgh, Churchill Livingstone

Sawyer C (1997) The mature child – how solicitors decide. *Family Law* **27**: 19–21

Smith K (1997) Too much, much too young. *Health Visitor* **20**(4): 137–8

Stone P (1995) *Road to Divorce*. Milton Keynes, Open University Press

United Nations (1948) General Assembly Resolution 217 (iii) UN Document A1810; article 71. Geneva, United Nations

Walton P (1997) The guardian ad litem's independence. *Family Law* **27**: 106–8

Weller B (1997) *Baillière's Nurses' Dictionary* (22nd edn). London, Baillière Tindall

Young A (1992) *Case Studies in Law and Nursing*. London, Chapman & Hall

Chapter 7 Mental handicap and mental health

Introduction

This chapter addresses the legal framework associated with mental handicap (learning disability) and mental illness. It must be stressed that these two groups of clients require very different care strategies, involving two separate nursing registrations and the involvement of specialist members of the multidisciplinary team. Despite this, the two groups of clients display broad similarities within the law and share some major ethical issues, one example being the capacity to give informed consent to treatment. The care of both groups is closely linked to social services provision as well as the care given by health professionals. The mentally handicapped and the mentally ill client also share, to some degree at least, a stigma in that, as the care of these groups of clients increasingly enters the community remit, media attention and poor publicity has resulted in further prejudicing them.

The term 'mental handicap' has been used as opposed to the current term of 'learning disability' in order to reflect the registration of nurses as Registered Nurse for the Mentally Handicapped (RNMH), and a major charitable voluntary body working within the area, MENCAP.

The chapter begins by considering the shared issues between the two groups of clients, although it must be emphasised that they are discrete groups within a broad framework and each client will present with individual needs, as would any other member of society.

The Mental Health Acts

The Mental Health Act 1983, relates wholly to England and Wales, with some similarities to Scotland, where the ruling statute is the Mental Health (Scotland) Act 1984. The Acts cover the compulsory admission to hospital of those clients often described as 'sectioned' as opposed to voluntary patients:

In practice, well over 90 per cent of those admitted to hospital suffering from mental illness or mental handicap are admitted as voluntary patients, although there are arguments that local authorities have not sufficiently used their powers to intervene to protect some of the most vulnerable and needy people in the community. (Fabb and Guthrie 1997, p. 202)

The underprovision of acute beds and facilities for the mentally ill is identified as a principal concern resulting from the rapid implementation of 'care in the community' policies.

Social policies and values have changed considerably during this century, and some consideration of the historical context is useful.

Legislation governing the treatment and care of the mentally ill dates back to before Victorian times; the 1834 Poor Law reformed the Tudor Poor Laws and recognised the needs of the sick pauper. The development of workhouse infirmaries threw together the physically ill, the mentally disordered and the mentally handicapped with little distinction between them, although these groups were normally segregated, the physically ill forming one group and the mentally ill and handicapped another. As these institutions grew, the perceived needs of the second group resulted in the passage of the 1845 Lunacy Act. The Lunacy Act was intended to regulate the newly created asylums, in which large numbers of people with mental illness or handicap were housed. As scientific knowledge progressed, it became clear that some distinction should be made between these two groups; the result was the Mental Deficiency Acts of 1913 and 1927 and the provision of institutions specifically to house those with mental handicap. Gates and Beacock (1997, p. 12) comment that 'This Act – the 1913 Act – introduced compulsory certification of "defectives" admitted to institutions. Clearly, this Act served to segregate people with a learning disability from the society at large.' The Mental Deficiency Acts provided originally for three categories of clients: the feeble minded, imbeciles and idiots.

The growth during the early twentieth century of the large mental asylums was only slightly affected by the Mental Treatment Act 1930, which made some provisions for outpatient care within the community. At this time, care of both the mentally handicapped and the mentally ill was principally by the local authority, with the costs of housing, treatment and care being met by the county rate-payers.

During the interwar years and continuing after 1945, many people were admitted to the asylums as 'moral defectives', a classification under the 1927 Mental Deficiency Act. Many others were admitted voluntarily to hospitals or other facilities without any apparent symptoms of mental illness or handicap. Some had minor mental illness; others were women who had become pregnant with an illegitimate child. This particular group remained, generally in mental hospitals, until the social policy of recent years discovered them. Sadly, many were too institutionalised to return fully to life in the community, so they remain in the hospitals to which they were committed in early adulthood. The plight of this group of people is given a memorial by an exclusion contained within the 1983 Mental Health Act. In the exclusion clause, promiscuity or immoral conduct is deemed to be outside the scope of the Act and does not constitute mental illness.

The hospitalised base of care reflected the importance of medical cure as opposed to social care, with the result that the institutions set up to house the mentally ill and handicapped continued with the inception of the NHS in 1948. The takeover by the NHS of the local authority sector encompassed that for mental handicap and mental health. This included those with an illness, as well as those with need for social care; this situation is only now changing.

The two strands of care, or as some commentators would say control, of the mentally ill and mentally handicapped continued until the 1959 Mental Health Act. 'The 1959 Act assimilated the law relating to mental handicap with that relating to mental illness, but was mental handicap – now generally known as learning disability – a medical problem at all?', questions Hoggett (1996, p. 1).

> If you have worked within a setting concerned with the care of mentally handicapped people, think about two or three clients.
>
> Did they require more social support or was the need for nursing care?
>
> What actions were needed to meet their needs?

The more social approach to both mental health and mental handicap is recognised in the Mental Health Act 1983, Part 1 of which sets out the meanings of mental disorder. The Act uses three terms to describe mental disorder: first, mental disorder, which includes mental illness, arrested or incomplete development of mind; second, severe mental impairment, defined as the severe impairment of intelligence and social functioning together with aggressive behaviour; and third, mental impairment, which also includes aggressive behaviour, but in which the mental impairment is not as severe as in the second classification. A fourth category, that of psychopathic disorder, is also included. A behavioural, as opposed to illness, approach allows both mentally handicapped and mentally ill clients to be included within the scope of the Act.

As discussed earlier, the vast majority of clients admitted to hospital-based care are classed as informal patients: they have been advised to enter hospital in order to receive care and are free to leave if they so wish. Thus these clients fall outside the Mental Health Acts.

Compulsory admission to hospital, often described as 'sectioning' a client under the Mental Health Act 1983 carries with it a number of checks and safeguards to ensure that the rights of the client are maintained as far as possible. As Dimond and Barker (1996, p. 72) discuss how 'Depriving individuals of their liberty is one of the greatest invasions of their rights. It is essential that there should be a clear appeal mechanism which is speedily and easily enforceable'. Sections 2, 3 and 4 of the Mental Health Act 1983 apply to the admission of clients. Section 2 relates to assessment of the client, and admission under the Section is for a maximum of 28 days and cannot be renewed. Section 3 concerns compulsory admission for treatment and lasts for a maximum of 6 months. Clients admitted under Section 2 may be transferred to Section 3 if assessment of their condition shows that a longer period of treatment is warranted. Section 4 admission is concerned with the emergency admission of a client for a maximum period of 72 hours. In all cases, record-keeping is essential, beginning with the completion of statutory forms by those making the application for admission. Application for admission may be made by the client's nearest relative, or an approved social worker and has to be agreed by one or more registered doctors according to which Section is appropriate. Record-keeping at ward or department level at the time of admission is also vital in order to assess the client's progress during admission.

Section 5 of the Mental Health Act 1983 is concerned with the detention of a client and its parts are referred to as holding orders. Under Section 5, a client may be detained for a maximum of 72 hours by the doctor in charge of the patient's treatment, while Section 5(4) allows a suitably qualified nurse to hold a client within the ward for a maximum of 6 hours, or 2 hours in Scotland. The clients held under the 'nurse's holding power' may be those admitted as informal patients but whose behaviours make them a potential danger to themselves or others. The nurse's authority to detain a client is only given to nurses with certain qualifications: the nurse must be registered on either Part 3 or 13 of the Register in the case of mental health nurses, or Part 5 or 15 for mental handicap nursing. In all cases, the patient must be informed of the holding order both verbally and in writing, and the managers must be informed. Statutory forms must also be completed in order to give a well-documented basis for the detention of the client.

In Scotland, the compulsory admission of a client is via two possible routes. Application may be made through the Sheriff Court under Section 18 of the Mental Health (Scotland) Act 1984, or there may be an emergency admission order under Section 24 of the Act. Admission orders under these Sections are for a maximum of 6 months or for 72 hours. The 72-hour order can be extended to 28 days.

As with the Mental Health Act 1983, application should be made, with the client's knowledge, by a mental health officer (MHO) who is a social worker, the equivalent to the English approved social worker, and the nearest relative. The application must also be supported by, as in England, a recommendation from two registered medical practitioners. In the situation when the client is so acutely mentally ill that immediate admission is desirable, an emergency admission order may be made by a doctor under Section 24 of the Act, following as far as is possible the procedure for admission under Section 18 as regards consent by the MHO and nearest relative.

Thinking point

> Are any of the clients whom you are caring for sectioned under either English or Scottish law?
>
> After obtaining permission from the ward/department manager, look at the patients' notes and see under which Section they were admitted.

As Dimond and Barker (1996, p. 72) outline, depriving a client of liberty is a serious matter, and the client has right of appeal built into the legislation. As with compulsory admission, the appeals process is also time related by the Mental Health Act 1983, clients being able to appeal against their admission to a Mental Health Review Tribunal. If the client does not appeal in person, the hospital will automatically make the appeal on the patient's behalf within 6 months of the Section being ordered, the case being reviewed at 3-yearly intervals thereafter. The Tribunal is made up of members drawn from not only the health care professions, but also legal and social services, who are able to examine the client's case objectively and discharge the client from the Section of the Act under which he or she has been detained. In some circumstances, the Tribunal is required to discharge clients, but this does not automatically mean the client's return to the community. Treatment may be continued as an informal patient instead of there being complete discharge into the community.

In England and Wales, the client's welfare is also monitored by the Mental Health Act Commission, set up under the Mental Health Act 1983. The Commission has a national membership of about 90 people who are appointed on a part-time 4-yearly basis by the Secretary of State. Commissioners have a particular remit in respect of clients under Section and are required to visit mental hospitals on an annual basis. On their visits, the Commissioners have the right to interview patients, check clients' records and inquire into any matter they wish relating to the sectioned clients.

The Secretary of State may authorise the visiting Commissioners to extend their remit to clients being treated on a voluntary basis.

In Scotland, rights of appeal are also built into the Mental Health Act (Scotland) 1984, being made to the Mental Welfare Commission. The Mental Welfare Commission has wide-ranging powers that include both hearing a case for discharge and investigation into the conditions in which mentally ill clients are held. It is made up of members from the medical and legal professions, together with lay representatives. Whereas the English Commissioners are appointed for a period of 4 years and are part time, the Scottish Commissioners include full-time members. The client may appeal to the Commission 28 days after admission, although, as Fabb and Guthrie state, 'It should be noted that there is no right of appeal against a sheriff's decision to admit the patient to hospital or against an emergency recommendation' (1997, p. 207). However, this does not totally preclude the client's rights to appeal against the admission, which in Scotland is closely linked to the mechanisms for appeal against sentence by a court (Ashton and Ward 1992, p. 96).

The Mental Health Acts are also concerned with the treatment and care of mentally ill offenders and the appropriateness of detaining those with mental health disorders in prisons. The needs of these groups, whether mentally handicapped or mentally ill, are met by both high-security special hospitals and medium secure units forming part of the local hospital provision for the mentally ill or handicapped. Caring for clients within these areas is a highly specialised form of care, and those who work in them have specialised skills and knowledge to meet the particular challenges of these groups.

Working with clients who are admitted to hospital or care against their will, particularly where treatment is required, requires health care professionals to act as advocates for their clients and highlights vital ethical issues. Skilled communication with those whose capacity to comprehend is limited is a key feature of work with these vulnerable groups, and the client should still have as full an understanding of their case as possible. While this is important for the compulsorily detained client, it is equally important for informal clients to be as fully aware of their treatment and care as is possible and reasonable.

Issues of confidentiality may be called into question, as the professionals may work together with voluntary organisations who represent the client.

Record-keeping forms a vital part of the care of the compulsorily detained client; the relevance of timing is important given the requirements of the Sections of the Mental Health Acts under which clients are admitted. Behavioural patterns that the client displays need to be identified, as do their interactions with others around them. The response of the client to drug therapy is also an important feature of record-keeping. To give an example, a client taking lithium, a drug with a narrow therapeutic range, requires regular blood-testing to monitor the blood level of the medication. The timing of the blood-testing is important, weekly blood tests being required initially and levels being monitored 3-monthly once blood levels are adequate. 'Every patient taking lithium should have a lithium card' (Downie *et al.* 1995, p. 133); the client must understand not only the need to carry the card, but also the interactions of lithium with other medications, some of which – such as low-dose, non-steroidal drugs, for example ibuprofen – may be purchased over the counter from a chemist. Ibuprofen is now widely advertised in the media as a treatment for headaches and minor viral illnesses but is liable to increase the level of lithium in the bloodstream, rendering the client more likely to suffer from unpleasant side-effects.

Consent to treatment

Consent to treatment is an important ethical issue within mental handicap and mental health care. Only the minority of clients who are admitted or detained under the Mental Health Act 1983 or Scottish legislation may be compulsorily treated. Consent to treatment by clients admitted on an informal basis would need to be sought in the usual way. Considerably more complex is the situation in which a mentally handicapped or mentally ill client is required to give consent to treatment for a physical condition. Hoggett (1996, p. 133) advises that:

The common law normally respects the right of any person to decide what shall be done with his own body. Thus any action which involves the use or the threat of force, however slight, upon his person will amount to a tort (and often also to a crime) unless there is consent or some other legal justification for acting without it.

A tort, broadly speaking, is that harm caused to a person without a justifiable reason and is actionable under civil law (see Chapter 1). Despite the fact that the treatment may be therapeutic, the fact that it has been undertaken without informed consent may constitute assault – the threat of force – or battery when the force is applied. When seeking consent to treatment therefore, the doctor will need to establish the competence of the client to give consent to what is proposed. In urgent cases, the doctor may have to work in the client's best interests, treatment being judged on the basis of the 'Bolam test'. In this test, named after a legal decision made in 1957, the doctor must decide whether the treatment would be 'accepted as proper by a responsible body of medical opinion' (Hoggett 1996, p. 137). In more difficult cases, where the client is unable to give consent, a guardian may be appointed, through the courts, to make decisions, including those about medical treatment, on behalf of the client.

Guardianship and the Court of Protection

Guardianship forms part of private law in both England and Scotland. Private law is that which affects the individual person in day-to-day living. A client who is unable to make major, everyday decisions, for example on financial matters, 'owing to his youth or his mental capacity, requires to have a guardian to act on his behalf' (Marshall 1995, p. 159). The Mental Health Acts of both England and Scotland make provision for those who are either mentally handicapped or mentally ill to have a guardian to preserve their interests and supervise their care. The guardian, once appointed, may be a relative or a social worker. For mentally handicapped or mentally ill clients whose conditions are such that they are unable to take care of their own affairs for the foreseeable future, the procedure·involves applying to the Court of Protection or Sheriff Court. Application to the Court is made by the nearest relative and an approved social worker (or MHO) and supported by medical recommendation in a fashion similar to that of applications for compulsory admission or treatment.

Guardianship shows a number of differences to compulsory admission under the English or Scottish Mental Health Acts in that the client does not have to be hospitalised or receive compulsory treatment. The place of residence must be stated on the order, and access to the client must be given to a doctor, the approved social worker or others, for example voluntary organisations representing the client's rights. Otherwise, the client is free to live as normal a life as possible.

Montgomery (1997, p. 315) states that 'Often the social services department will be the guardian, but it is possible for a private person to be the guardian.' This allows relatives or suitable others, once appointed, to take charge of the client's affairs, including financial matters. Review of the guardianship arrangements is built into the statutes in order to prevent abuse of the client.

Thinking point

Do you care for a client group that includes clients who have a guardian?

If you do, try to talk to the appointed guardian about their role in the patient's affairs. If the guardian is a relative of the client, discuss your approach to them first with the key worker or manager.

Abuse of the client

One of the purposes of the appointment of a guardian to manage the client's affairs is to prevent abuse, in particular financial abuse of the client's assets. Financial abuse may range from outright theft or misappropriation of the client's assets to misuse of social security benefits to which he or she is entitled. However, guardianship only applies to a minority of clients with mental handicap or mental health conditions; the majority will either manage their own affairs with some degree – or not – of supervision or will nominate an agent. An agent is usually a member of the client's own family who is able to collect social security benefits on the client's behalf.

The mentally handicapped and the mentally ill are as liable to other forms of abuse as any other dependent group. Both physical and sexual abuse may result in criminal proceedings being taken against the abuser. This highlights the difficulties of gaining evidence against the accused in order for the Crown Prosecution Service to bring the case to court. The Police and Criminal Evidence Act 1984 (PACE 1984) takes special note of the needs of potential witnesses, whether the prosecution be for abuse or any other crime. PACE 1984 is another example of how clients with either mental handicap or mental illness are treated as one group with special needs during a police investigation: 'For the most part, the Act and Codes treat the mentally disordered and mentally handicapped in a similar way, although the problems suffered by each stem from significantly different causes' (Lidstone and Palmer 1996, p. 488). The 'Codes' are codes of practice that accompany the PACE 1984 and give the police guidelines on how to act in given situations. The code of practice requires that, when a police officer wishes to question a client, an 'appropriate adult' must be present. An 'appropriate adult' is one as defined in the code of practice, Section C, and it is preferable that he or she is known to the client in order to protect the client's interests during interview, although this cannot always be the case. The 'appropriate adult' may be the client's guardian or a relative, or someone who has expertise in the care and treatment of mentally disordered clients. Alternatively, the 'appropriate adult' may be a health care professional/worker or a social worker who will accompany the client during interview. During the interview, the 'appropriate adult' will act as the client's advocate in order to ensure that the client is not pressurised or led during questioning. Should the client be an accused person, he or she has the same rights to legal representation as any other person. A similar framework exists for the interviewing of child witnesses by the police.

Not in my backyard...

Care in the community for people with mental handicap or mental illness has always been a controversial issue. Social policy for the mentally handicapped and mentally ill has followed a pattern similar to that for the elderly in long-stay institutions, and it is not proposed to repeat material given in other chapters of this book. However, the ethical dimension is one that can be used to examine the issues, especially in the light of media publicity given to acts of violence by a tiny minority of clients and the stigma popularly attributed to mental handicap and mental health. This portion of the chapter refers to the vast majority of clients who are not sectioned under the Mental Health Act 1983 or the Mental Health (Scotland) Act 1984. Provision of care in the community refers to both local authority provision and that provided by the voluntary organisations and the private sector.

The four major ethical principles of autonomy, beneficence, non-maleficence and justice that Beauchamp and Childress (1994) consider to underpin health care can be used to illustrate a discussion on care in the community. As with any debate of an ethical nature, there are two sides to every argument.

The first is from the client's point of view. Personal autonomy, to live as one pleases, is a fundamental human right:

Human rights are moral rights of a very important kind, shared equally by all persons. These human rights are the union of two kinds of rights; self-determination or liberty rights and rights to be cared for or well-being rights. (Bandman and Bandman 1995, p. 92)

The long-stay pattern of care provision denied, in a large part, clients' right to autonomy over much of their lives. Limited autonomy was possible in minor decision-making, but the major choices that most of us take for granted, such as choosing where and how to live, when and where to take a holiday, and what food to buy and eat, were not available to residents in long-stay care facilities. Removal into the community restored the principle, at least in theory, of the client's human right to care being preserved by the employment of carers living or working in small community-based homes run on a family model. The development of small homes within the community is a particular feature of community care of the mentally handicapped, a number of houses often being grouped together.

The ethical principle of beneficence can also be addressed, together with its broad opposite, non-maleficence. The 'principle of beneficence refers to a moral obligation to act for the benefit of others' (Beauchamp and Childress 1994, p. 260). To allow autonomy, albeit with support from paid carers, to a disadvantaged sector of the community must be a move to which most people would subscribe. To facilitate the move into the community, many hospitals developed extensive rehabilitation programmes to give their clients the best chance of the maximum independence that they could achieve. Staff were relocated or recruited to work in the new smaller, community-based homes, and new day centres developed to allow rehabilitation and treatment to continue within the specialised needs of the client group. Non-maleficence is the prevention of harm, in the case of health care to the clients who are receiving care. In terms of care in the community, this can mean the provision of safe housing, adherence to health and safety issues, and the continuation of care and rehabilitation, allowing individuals to reach their maximum potential. In some places, health care workers will have to make decisions on behalf of clients who are not capable of personal autonomy, and observance of the principles of beneficence and non-maleficence will feature as they act as advocates for the client. As Singleton and McLaren observe, 'It might be argued that really we only have one principle here and that promoting well-being and not harming just represent opposite ends of a continuum' (1995, p. 40).

Thinking point

> Think of a client whom you have cared for who is not fully able to make autonomous decisions. (This is often described as being mentally incompetent.)
>
> How were decisions made on the client's behalf? Was one key worker involved, or were others consulted?

The fourth principle, that of justice, is generally held to go beyond the client as a person and to focus on the wider issues that, although they may affect an individual, are the wider issues of resource management and the provision of care. While long-stay hospitals were a relatively cheap form of care for those who required it, individualised care in the community is comparatively expensive. As described earlier in this chapter, care of the mentally handicapped in particular only became part of the NHS because of a quirk of history as the NHS was formed. Restoring this client group to the community has required a huge investment on the part of society as a whole.

Every argument has two sides. To health care workers and professionals, the benefit of care within the community, except in cases of severe illness or in an acute episode, is a fairly logical progression from institutionalised care. Sadly, not everyone sees it that way, and as care moved into the community, the 'not in my backyard' reaction began. People who were very happy to consider community care as appropriate were suddenly less happy when they found that a home was planned within their area. In a democratic country such as the UK, applications for planning permission or change of use of property made to the local authority are a matter of public record, the nearest neighbours being contacted by the council concerned. The neighbours have a right to object to the proposed building or change of use of an existing building and may give, as the grounds for their objection, the effect that the development might have on property values in the area. High levels of media attention given to the murder of Jonathan Zito by Christopher Clunis, a mentally ill man, and a number of similar cases increased the fears of many members of the public concerning the mentally ill and mentally handicapped being housed in the community.

Thinking point

> Using the four major principles of ethics – autonomy, beneficence, non-maleficence and justice – consider the arguments that might be put forward by neighbours when a community home for mentally ill people is planned for their area.
>
> How do you think these concerns could be overcome?

Although the arguments concerning community care are far from over, successive governments have endorsed the concept. What has become apparent is an underprovision of safe care for mental health patients suffering an acute episode and a desperate need for more mental health beds in many areas of the country. Despite these problems, the clear focus of the two NHS White Papers *The New NHS: Modern, Dependable* (Department of Health 1997) and *Designed to Care: Renewing the National Health Service in Scotland* (Scottish Office 1997) is to continue to invest in care delivery within the community.

References and further reading

Ashton G and Ward A (1992) *Mental Handicap and the Law*. London, Sweet & Maxwell

Bandman E and Bandman B (1995) *Nursing Ethics through the Life Span*. Englewood Cliffs. NJ, Prentice-Hall

Barker P (1997) *Assessment in Psychiatric and Mental Health Nursing: In Search of the Whole Person.* Cheltenham, Stanley Thornes

Beauchamp T and Childress J (1994) *Principles of Biomedical Ethics* (4th edn). Oxford, Oxford University Press

Cambridge P, Hayes L and Knapp M (1994) *Care in the Community: Five Years On.* Aldershot, Arena

Department of Health (1997) *The New NHS: Modern, Dependable.* London, HMSO

Dimond B and Barker F (1996) *Mental Health Law for Nurses.* Oxford, Blackwell Science

Downie G, Mackenzie J and Williams A (1995) *Pharmacology and Drug Management for Nurses.* Edinburgh, Churchill Livingstone

Fabb J and Guthrie T (1997) *Social Work Law in Scotland.* Edinburgh, Butterworth

Gates B and Beacock C (eds) (1997) *Dimensions of Learning Disability.* London, Baillière Tindall

Hoggett B (1996) *Mental Health Law* (4th edn). London, Sweet & Maxwell

Jones K (1993) *Asylums and After: A Revised History of the Mental Health Services from the Early 18th Century to the 1990s.* London, Athlone Press

Lidstone K and Palmer C (1996) *Bevan and Lidstone's The Investigation of Crime: A Guide to Police Powers* (2nd edn). London, Butterworth

Marshall E (1995) *General Principles of Scots Law* (6th edn). Edinburgh, W Green/Sweet & Maxwell

Montgomery J (1997) *Health Care Law.* Oxford, Oxford University Press

Scottish Office (1997) *Designed to Care: Renewing the National Health Service in Scotland.* Edinburgh, Stationery Office

Scull A (1979) *Museums of Madness: The Social Organisation of Insanity in Nineteenth-Century England.* Harmondsworth, Penguin

Seabrooke S and Sprack J (1996) *Criminal Evidence and Procedure: The Statutory Framework.* London, Blackstone Press

Singleton J and McLaren S (1995) *Ethical Foundations of Health Care: Responsibilities in Decision Making.* London, CV Mosby

Titterton M (ed.) (1994) *Caring for People in the Community: The New Welfare.* London, Jessica Kingsley

Chapter 8 The dying client

Introduction

Caring for people when the end of their life is approaching combines many of the legal, moral and ethical debates of our time. The rise of the hospice movement, the acceptance of the idea of death with dignity and the care of the dying as a speciality have all made their contribution to legal and ethical issues related to the dying client. In this chapter, some of the legal issues relating to the care of the dying are outlined and broadly related to the care situation. As medical science advances, a thin line is developing between those who are being prevented from dying and those who are being prevented from living, creating a legal and ethical maze for health care personnel. It is also necessary to consider the situation of those who have attempted to take their own life and the attitude of the law towards suicide.

Euthanasia

Euthanasia is a word derived from classical Greek and is defined as 'an easy or good death'; it is more commonly used to mean 'the deliberate ending of life of a person suffering from an incurable disease' (Weller 1997, p. 152).

In modern health care, euthanasia has become one of the controversial issues of our time, being closely linked to the law of homicide. Both murder and manslaughter come under the umbrella title of 'homicide' and can affect the ways in which care is delivered to terminally ill patients. One definition of murder is that 'there must be an unlawful killing of a human being under the Queen's peace with malice aforethought the victim dying within a year and a day' (Keenan 1995, p. 512). It is possible then that the prescription and administration of lethal drugs or substances, if given deliberately to end the client's life, could be liable to investigation as murder. A slightly lesser offence under the law is termed 'manslaughter' and is divided into two areas: voluntary and involuntary. Voluntary manslaughter relies on the presence of provocation or diminished responsibility at the time of the offence. Involuntary manslaughter is when the client dies as a result of an act done intentionally but not necessarily with the aim of causing death. Involuntary manslaughter may also be a result of gross negligence on the part of health care professionals, although 'a very high degree of negligence is necessary for the establishment of a crime' (Keenan 1995, p. 515).

The laws of homicide are fundamentally linked to the care of the terminally ill patient; although professional interests have emphasised the care of cancer patients, it is important to acknowledge that the care of those with any other terminal illness – or indeed old age – is no exception to the law. Health care professionals may not give a lethal substance that would bring about the client's death, but ever stronger drugs may be prescribed to alleviate pain and distress. Dimond (1995, p. 254) outlines the situation:

The position is clear for professional staff. Even though they sympathise with a patient's wish to die, they are prohibited by the criminal law in taking any steps or giving any advise to the patient to help him carry out this wish.

The treatment and care of those with a terminal illness often involves high doses of pain-killing drugs – analgesics – the storage and prescription of which are covered by the Misuse of Drugs Act 1971 and its most recent Regulations. Drugs named in the Schedules of the Regulations are often described as 'controlled' drugs and are the drugs implicated in addiction and abuse, although they are used therapeutically for the control of severe pain. Regulations concerning these drugs are stringent in terms of their storage, their administration and the associated record-keeping. In hospitals, these drugs are kept in a locked cupboard inside another locked cupboard, the keys to which are held by the registered nurse in charge of the ward. The situation in the community will be dependent on the setting in which care is being delivered, for example a nursing home where security for medicines will resemble that of the hospital, or the client's own home where such measures may not be possible. In a nursing home, the registered nurse in charge at the time will be responsible for all drugs including the controlled drugs, and the nurse's actions are governed both by the Misuse of Drugs Act 1971 (1985 Regulations) and the UKCC *Code of Professional Conduct* (1992) in the same way as for a nurse employed in a hospital.

Thinking point

> Which drugs might be used when a client is in severe pain?
>
> How are they stored in your place of work?
>
> How are they recorded and accounted for?

Clients who have suffered trauma or devastating brain damage may require ventilation as part of their care. In this treatment, the ventilator takes the part of the client's respiratory system in order for the body to receive sufficient oxygen for its physical needs; this is often termed 'life support'. Relatives and the health care team may be faced with the difficult dilemma of whether the machine should be turned off and the client allowed to die, and in this situation the law, through examination of individual cases, has developed a format as a guide to those caring for the client. There are broadly two situations in which life support systems may be discontinued. The first is if the patient, after careful testing, is shown to be brain dead. Two doctors must conduct the tests, one of whom should be the consultant who has been treating the client, the second another experienced doctor. They test the basic reflexes originating in the brain stem (hence 'brain stem death'), reflexes affecting the eyes, the respiratory reflexes and functions that are essential to life. The second situation occurs if the patient's probable long-term outcome is very poor. Then, even if the patient can breathe unaided after ventilation has been discontinued, the machine need not be restarted should the patient relapse; alernatively, ventilation may not be attempted at all.

The first part of this section rested on the law relating to health care professionals working with terminally ill clients. Central to the concept of euthanasia are the clients and their wishes. Although the relatives and carers legally have no rights in the decision-making, they may play a large part in the communication of the client's wishes to others. Knowing what the client's own wishes are may help health care professionals to make a decision about what may be done in the client's best interests. Indeed, the carers' advice on the client's care may well be sought by the professional team and prove to be invaluable. There is, however, the problem of the relatives and carers having a vested interest, either physically or emotionally, in the survival or demise of the client. As in all other areas of care, dying clients must have choice over their treatment and be able to take part in the planning of care or have their wishes met whenever possible. The meeting of the clients' wishes in the period leading up to their death falls within palliative care: 'When the doctors responsible for the patient confess that nothing more can be done to reverse the process of his illness, palliative care begins' (Kenworthy *et al.* 1992, p. 315). The interval between this point and the death of the client may be either short or long, in some cases years, with distressing symptoms, as opposed to the underlying illness, receiving treatment.

The hospice movement founded by Dr Cicely Saunders at St Christopher's Hospice in London is the leader in the field of palliative care and the relief of distressing symptoms. Pain, and the relief of pain using high dosages of analgesics, forms much of the work of the hospice staff, who are often willing to advise health care professionals on the therapeutic uses of drugs used not only in pain relief, but also in the control of other distressing symptoms. Hospices are registered with the local authority as nursing homes under Part 2 of the Registered Nursing Homes Act 1984 and funded by a combination of sources. Local authority and health authority grants, together with local fundraising efforts, combine to aid the client who has a life-shortening illness for whom palliative care is the most appropriate option. Care of the client within a hospice demands the skills of many professional groups and is not confined to medicine and nursing: the multi-disciplinary team may include radiotherapists, those concerned with the spiritual and psychological care of the dying client as well as complementary therapists.

As with any phase of health care, the client has a right to accept or refuse therapy or treatment. The underlying legal position is currently governed by the Suicide Act 1961, which removed suicide from the criminal law structure and made it legally acceptable for clients to refuse treatment even though that refusal could result in their death. However, Section 2 of the Suicide Act clearly outlines the penalties for any person who assists in procuring a suicide, with a maximum term of imprisonment of up to 14 years should they be found guilty.

The Suicide Act 1961 bought the client and the professional more closely into the developing and still evolving debate on euthanasia and its legal underpinning. The Act began the clarification process in respect of the legal standing of professionals caring for clients who have decided that they wish only symptomatic treatment.

Advance directives (living wills)

The advance directive is likely to play an important part in the care of the terminally ill in the future, although it is important to state that an advance directive may only be written by those who have reached the legal age of majority, which is 18 years of age in the UK. The directive can also be withdrawn by the client at any time and should be regularly reviewed in the light of medical developments. The advance directive is increasingly being recognised as a valid document in civil law, although any order to end life remains outside the law. Health care professionals and workers are obliged to treat the client according to his wishes. Active euthanasia (the health care team deliberately bringing about the client's death) cannot be included, but passive euthanasia may be contained within the refusal of treatment and form part of the advance directive. It is important to emphasise that patients have, at any time, the right to refuse treatment or medication, but this refusal, along with the reason for it, should be carefully recorded by the care staff on each occasion.

A Legal Framework for Caring

Thinking point

> Have you ever cared for a client who has refused drug treatment of any sort?
>
> How often did he or she refuse it, and was the reason for refusal noted?
>
> How was the refusal/reason documented?

Greater media attention to medical matters has increased public awareness of the options available in what was previously the domain of health care. Increasing knowledge may affect relationships and care delivery as patients become more educated and assertive about what they want. The Patients Association advises that:

The purpose of an advance statement is to let people know your preferences about the future medical treatment you would like to have or wish to refuse if you are in a condition which prevents you from making your views known. (Patients Association 1996, p. 8).

Importantly, within this view is the idea that the client can opt in or out of treatments that are (or are not) acceptable to them. The idea of opting in or out of treatment implies that the client is able to make that decision – is mentally competent – and has the necessary knowledge to make a judgement. Although it is not essential in common law, the client should be advised to seek the fullest advice before writing an advance directive and, wherever possible, to have it witnessed by a medical practitioner who knows the client in order to establish mental competence at the time of making the directive.

Despite the fact that relatives have little legal status, the making of an advance directive may include the nomination of a 'health care proxy', often a relative or a close friend whom the client has chosen to act on their behalf: 'You must ensure that you have told this person what you would find acceptable or unacceptable' (Patients Association 1996, p. 9). The legal basis for advance directives is principally case law, which is currently decided on an individual basis, but the general trend is to support the patient's and relatives' wishes when they are known.

As the law related to advance directives is evolving, draft legislation proposed by the Law Commission on Mental Incapacity (Law Commission 231), which included a section on advance directives, has been postponed by the 1997 general election. Since the election, the incoming government has stated its interest in reviewing the Law Commission report with a view to instituting legislation. Despite this, the acceptance in common law of advance directives places a responsibility on care staff to meet the patient's wishes when they are known. In order to meet these requirements, the care team must maintain high levels of communication between themselves and with their client.

The multidisciplinary team in practice

The importance of communication among the multiprofessional team is stressed within the codes of conduct or rules of the individual professions. The *Rules of Professional Conduct for Occupational Therapists* state that 'Occupational Therapists shall consult and co-operate with those with whom they come into contact during the course of their professional duties' and this is echoed by the *Rules of Professional Conduct for Physiotherapists*: 'Chartered Physiotherapists shall communicate and co-operate with other health and allied professionals and all others caring for the patient in the interests of the patient.' The UKCC states, in Paragraphs 5 and 6 of its *Code of Professional Conduct*, that their practitioners shall 'Work in an open and co-operative manner with patients, clients and their families... foster their independence and recognise and respect their involvement in the planning and delivery of care', and that they should 'Work in a collaborative and co-operative manner with health care professionals and others involved in providing care, and recognise and respect their particular contributions within the health care team.' The English text of the *International Code of Medical Ethics* reads, 'A PHYSICIAN SHALL in all types of medical practice, be dedicated to providing competent medical service in full technical and moral independence with compassion and respect for human dignity' (all cited by Singleton and McLaren 1995, pp. 176, 172, 170 and 165 respectively).

The rules and codes of conduct are an important guide for all health care professionals and should also shape the behaviour and thinking of those in training to qualify for the professions. Unqualified staff are not bound by the codes but should be encouraged by their supervisors to maintain the standards set by the statutory bodies governing the professionals. For trainee members, many of the professions have developed modified student codes as a guideline. Strictly speaking, the rules and codes of conduct are codes of ethics that have been developed by the individual registering bodies but provide guidelines for the law to judge the conduct expected of professionals under the legal duty of care.

Care of the client at the end of life demands the skills of a large number of professional groups, many of whom work both on a curative as well as a palliative basis. Multidisciplinary team therapy professionals may include hospital-based radiologists and radiographers who specialise in the treatment of cancer and the control of distressing symptoms using X-rays (radiotherapy) and radio-isotopes. Doctors and nurses who specialise in pain control and palliative care may also work with the client and family in addition to the core team. Caring for the client's spiritual needs is also of vital importance to overall well-being, and spiritual guidance and support may well be given by a priest of the client's choosing.

Thinking point

> Consider one client whom you have been caring for. How many professionals are there within the care team?
>
> How does each profession record its input? Are records held jointly by the professions, or does each profession keep a separate record?

The importance of good record-keeping is paramount, oral communication being insufficient in the event of client deterioration. A written record is vital for communication to continue effectively and to ensure that, in the event of a later enquiry, the actions of team members are clearly recorded.

The sensitivity of caring for a client and family while the client is in the terminal stages of illness, especially where the client has determined his or her own treatment, may give rise to issues of conscientious objection within the care team. This may be especially true where active treatment for the primary condition is being discontinued. There is no right in law for refusal of care in this situation, and nursing staff in particular must continue care for the alleviation of pain and for the client's basic needs. However, this is a difficult circumstance and the rules and codes request that care staff with a conscientious objection should discuss this with their qualified supervisor in order to effect a solution to their plight.

Conscientious objection is a particularly pertinent issue for nursing staff in that the provision of food and water forms part of nursing care. An example of this is given by the case of Tony Bland, who lived in a persistent vegetative state and was fed and hydrated by use of a nasogastric tube. In 1993, the Bland family took the case to court, requesting that treatment to keep him alive should be withdrawn. Their wish was granted as Tony had no chance of recovery, and Airedale NHS Trust was ordered to cease what was essentially nursing care only. This placed the nursing staff, as employees of the Trust, in a difficult situation in that they had to withdraw water, placing them in a moral dilemma in which the law opposed what was, to many, a basic right.

Physician-assisted suicide and double effect

Within the framework of, and closely allied to, advance directives is the determination of a few clients suffering from terminal illness to die at a time of their own choosing. As discussed earlier within this chapter, health care professionals are clearly and legally forbidden from acting in any way that could deliberately shorten the client's life. This may place doctors – who do the prescribing – as well as nurses, the principal group administering drugs, in a difficult situation as many of the drugs prescribed as death is approaching may also have the effect of shortening life. The doctor must then weigh up the advantages to the client of the prescription against the potential harmful effects of the drug. This is known as the 'double effect': the beneficial effects of the drug being outweighed by the possibility of reducing the client's already short life expectation.

In a few areas in the world – although not in the UK – legal frameworks have been developed that permit clients to bring about their own death by the use of computer programmes linked to a lethal drug dose that has been prescribed by a medical practitioner.

'Do not resuscitate' orders

This section of the chapter is concerned entirely with the care of clients who have a known diagnosis and whose illness is liable either to end in death or to severely and adversely affect their quality of life. A cardiac arrest affecting a previously healthy person is not discussed; the expectation of the law is clear cut – that they should be treated until it is obvious that they cannot survive the arrest.

A consideration with seriously ill clients, and one which is commonly encountered in hospitals, is whether or not cardiopulmonary resuscitation in the event of cardiac arrest is appropriate. The decision may have already been made by the client as part of an advance directive, in which case the client's wishes must be respected. Legal practice, and the recommendations of the Law Commission (1995) are that, in the absence of any other known instructions to the contrary, life-saving measures must be attempted. Thus emergency staff should commence resuscitation until evidence to the contrary in the form of a directive or the patient's clearly stated previous wishes is available.

Where it is unlikely that a client will survive a cardiac arrest, or the client's long-term prognosis is poor, a 'Do not resuscitate' (DNR) order may be decided on by the consultant in charge of the client's medical treatment. This decision should also be discussed with the relatives or next of kin, documented in the medical notes and conveyed to all those involved in the client's care. Good communication can forestall what Dimond (1995, p. 253) describes as the 'no-win' situation that exists for care staff:

She [the nurse] may feel that she is an impossible no-win situation: if she does not initiate resuscitation procedures following a collapse, then she could possibly be criticised by relatives or even face criminal charges; if, on the other hand she ignores the letters NFR [not for resuscitation] and starts resuscitation procedures, then she could be criticised by the medical staff and face disciplinary proceedings.

Record-keeping is a feature of the rules and codes of conduct for all qualified professionals, and this is one of the many situations when it is essential, especially when there is disagreement among the team over how the patient should be treated.

Despite the fact that relatives have no strict legal standing in the decision-making, their views and feelings on the subject may often be sought and require sensitive handling by care staff: they may be the only way in which the client's views may be made known to the care team. Although relatives may influence the decision of whether or not resuscitation should be carried out, it is important to realise that, at this time, it is the medical prognosis and the likelihood of recovery that will be the principal deciders in the case. Some acknowledgment should also be given to the ethical dimensions of such a decision: 'There are tremendous difficulties in determining whether or not an individual's life is worth living' (Singleton and McLaren 1995, p. 69). Regular review of DNR orders is crucial, with each review carefully documented in the client's notes, the review period being dependent on the client's condition. This is important as the client's health status changes and either improves or deteriorates. The ethical and humanitarian effects on relatives of the DNR decision may also need to be considered. Relatives may require considerable support before, during and after the death to prevent feelings of guilt about a decision that they have influenced on their loved one's behalf. In some cases, the client may have nominated a 'health care proxy' to assist in the decision-making and advise professionals of the client's wishes.

Following on from the decision for a DNR order and its documentation are the legal principles underlying the decision in relation to the order. The tort of battery – a tort being 'a civil wrong which entitles a person who is injured by its commission to claim damages for his loss, whether purely by way of reparation or as a way of bringing home to the defendant the anti-social nature of his act' (Shears and Stephenson 1996, p. 303) – could be involved if the client were resuscitated against his expressed wishes. Importantly, battery can also arise from a failure or omission to act and may constitute negligence on the part of the professional. Scottish law does not recognise battery, using instead the term 'assault' to cover these offences, the extent of which are defined by the body of common law in Scotland. The difficulties of the situation emphasise the importance of accurate and careful record-keeping if the health care team are not to risk legal proceedings. It must be remembered, however, in caring for clients at the end of their life, that they are likely to die from their previously diagnosed illness and that the probable outcome of the illness plays a big part in the decision-making. In all likelihood, the majority of clients will not even be considered for cardiopulmonary resuscitation as they will probably die without any cardiac condition demanding resuscitation; this is an essential concept in the care of the dying.

Thinking point

> Are you caring for a client who is 'Not for resuscitation'?
>
> Who made the decision and how is the decision recorded?
>
> Are you able to find out about what discussion went into the decision-making?

A far more difficult ethical and moral area arises within resuscitation of the very elderly client. The elderly are reaching the natural end of life, and this special circumstance should not be lost in the general arguments relating to younger clients. Elderly clients and their carers are subject to exactly the same legal framework as others. In a number of hospitals, it is now routine practice, backed by formal hospital policy, to discuss with elderly clients, on their admission, their wishes with regard to resuscitation. This approach requires tact and sensitivity on the part of all staff and documentation of the outcome by a consultant or registrar in the medical notes, along with suitable review dates. This approach allows for more clarity for the legal issues in that a decision is made and documented for the team to work with.

After death

When the client has died, there are still ethical and legal issues to consider. The immediate care of the relatives or friends of the deceased client is a high priority and needs sensitive handling. They are often very distressed or display other signs of stress, such as anger against care staff. Should the client have known religious beliefs, these need to be complied with and the body treated with respect and dignity, any property being carefully handled and accounted for in order that it may be returned to the next of kin.

Many employers have developed guidelines and policies to help with the care of the body. Occasionally, the body must be left as it was at death – if the cause of death is unknown, if death resulted from trauma or if a post mortem is necessary in law. In such cases, the body, without being washed or cleaned, is removed to the mortuary, leaving medical equipment such as intravenous cannulae and catheters in place. The need to leave medical equipment in situ should be discussed sensitively with the relatives, who may wish to see the body after death, remembering that they are undergoing the devastating event of a sudden bereavement.

The UK has become a country with a significant number of ethnic and cultural minorities. The welfare of the dying client may well involve meeting spiritual needs that are unfamiliar to the health care worker: 'A nurse may, for example, be supporting a bereaved family. Here respect for autonomy necessarily entails balancing the wishes of different individuals together, and having regard for the family as a whole' (Cribb 1995, p. 27). For example, a dying Muslim:

may wish to sit or lie with his face towards Mecca, and moving the bed if necessary to make this possible will be appreciated. Another Muslim, usually a relative, may whisper the call to prayer into the dying person's ear, and family members may recite prayers around the bed. (Green 1991, p. 2)

Other religions – Judaism and Hinduism – prefer the body to be touched as little as possible and for last offices to be performed by family members or a specially appointed person.

Thinking point

Check whether your workplace has a policy or guideline for the care of the body after death (often described as 'laying out'). If so, read it.

Does the policy discuss the care of the body if the patient is of a non-Christian faith, or recommend how the carer may find out about the needs of other religions following death?

In some care settings, qualified nursing staff are permitted to verify – confirm – death in a client who is expected to die. This is not the same as certifying the death and may only be done by a nurse who has been given the authority of his or her employer so to do. A death certificate is a document completed by a doctor stating the cause of death, and then being taken, usually by the nominated next of kin, to the Registrar of Births and Deaths, in order that the death can be registered. The cause of death given on the death certificate becomes an anonymous part of the national mortality statistics. The registration process is governed by the Births and Deaths Registration Act 1953. Following some deaths, it may be necessary for a post mortem examination (or autopsy) to take place, and the written consent of the next of kin to be sought for this, often in order to advance understanding of the illness that has caused the death. In some circumstances, the death must be reported to the Coroner. 'At the present time, about a third of all deaths in England and Wales are reported to Coroners' (Dean 1996, p. 75), not all of which will result in a post mortem. In Scotland, the office equivalent to that of Coroner is held by the Procurator Fiscal as an extension of his role in the investigation and prosecution of crime.

When a death is reported to the Coroner or Procurator Fiscal, the death cannot be registered until the cause of death is agreed. Campbell (1997, pp. 53–4) summarises the reasons for referral to the Coroner:

All violent, unnatural or suspicious deaths
All deaths without obvious cause
All deaths where the deceased had not been seen by a doctor in the two weeks before death
All deaths occurring during a surgical procedure
All deaths caused by industrial poisoning
All deaths of persons in custody of the police or prison service.

The Scottish office of Procurator Fiscal is held by appointment from the Lord Advocate's office. In England, the work of the Coroner is covered by the Coroners Act 1988, much of the administration of the department being carried out by the Coroner's Officer or Officers. The Coroner, or Officers, will explain their work to doctors and other health care staff and advise on specific cases when requested to do so by registered staff.

Transplantation

A major issue especially following the unexpected death of a younger client may be that of the transplantation of donor organs. Where the victim of an accident or sudden illness is an adult and is carrying an organ donor card, the consent to donation is relatively straightforward. However, as outlined in the preceding section, many who meet this type of death will be liable to notification to the Coroner; this will be a matter of great urgency if the organs are to be suitable for transplantation. Where the wishes of the victim are known in advance, or the next of kin agree to organ donation, the Human Tissue Act 1961 – the first of three statutes governing transplantation – rules that the Coroner's permission must also be obtained prior to the harvest of organs if there is a likelihood of a post mortem or inquest into the death. This permission is obtained on an emergency, fast-procedure basis if transplantation is being considered.

The Corneal Tissue Act 1986 allows either medical practitioners or others who have been trained in the technique to remove the eyes of deceased persons for use in transplant. This can, of course, only happen once permission has been granted either prior to death by the client, or by their relatives, in the same way as applies to other organs. This Act governing transplantation is specifically directed at corneal transplant – the cornea being the 'transparent portion of the anterior surface of the eyeball' (Weller 1997, p. 105).

The development of transplantation, the improvement in drug therapy and the evolution of organ donation by living donors to people either related or not related to them led to the development of the Human Organ Transplants Act, which became law in 1989. The Act safeguards donors and recipients, providing for counselling and very strict record-keeping by health care professionals employed in the field of transplantation. The Act is supported by Regulations, which allow for a reasonably speedy legal response as the issues surrounding tissue transplants alter in the light of further research.

Conclusion

This chapter has considered some of the legal issues surrounding caring for the dying client and following death. The issues relating to euthanasia are clear cut: at the present time, no health care worker may act in a way that will deliberately end a client's life however sympathetic they may feel towards the client's plight. Despite this, the notion of 'physician-assisted suicide' is gaining ground and was hotly debated at the 1997 British Medical Association conference.

Dying people are a client group who are particularly vulnerable and for whom the law is evolving with respect to the acceptance of advance directives. Many health care professionals are opposed to advance directives on ethical grounds, while also subscribing to the philosophy of client autonomy, an internal conflict that will never be easily resolved.

The legal underpinning of DNR orders is clear and is essentially led by medical practitioners with support from the health care team. All members of the team will be involved in the care and support of this client group and the family and friends as the client approaches the end of life. Additional support may be given by chaplains and ministers of religion or bereavement counsellors with their own codes of ethics and practices.

In the situation of sudden or unexpected death, the Coroner and possibly the police may join the more usual members of the multiprofessional team. The work of these groups is also closely linked to the national legal framework.

Care of the client at the end of life is a demanding and frequently rewarding speciality in which the multiprofessional team needs to work closely together in order to support the client, their family and friends through what may be a very difficult time. As there are many legal and ethical issues, diverging opinions and input from those with specific expertise, good record-keeping is an essential feature in order to promote good-quality care and good communication, and to comply with legal demands.

References and further reading

Campbell K (1997) Post mortems: how and why they are carried out. *Nursing Times* **93**(16): 53–4

Cribb A (1995) The ethical dimension. In Tingle J and Cribb A (eds) *Nursing Law and Ethics*. Oxford, Blackwell Science, pp. 21–35

Dean P (1996) Death certification and the role of the coroner. In Payne-James J (ed.) *Medicolegal Essentials in Health Care*. Edinburgh, Churchill Livingstone, pp. 71–8

Dennis IH (1989) *Sweet & Maxwell's Criminal Law Statutes* (2nd edn). London, Sweet & Maxwell

Dimond B (1995) *Legal Aspects of Nursing.* Hemel Hempstead, Prentice-Hall

Green J (1991) *Death with Dignity: Meeting the Spiritual Needs of Patients in a Multicultural Society,* Vol. 1. London, Macmillan Magazines

Green J (1993) *Death with Dignity: Meeting the Spiritual Needs of Patients in a Multicultural Society,* Vol. 2. London, Macmillan Magazines

Keenan D (1995) *Smith and Keenan's English Law.* London, Pitman Publishing

Kenworthy N, Snowley S and Gilling C (1992) *Common Foundation Studies in Nursing.* Edinburgh, Churchill Livingstone

Law Commission (1995) *Mental Incapacity* (Part V). Law Commission No. 231. London, HMSO

Neuberger J (1994) *Caring for Dying People of Different Faiths* (2nd edn). London, CV Mosby

Patients Association (1996) *Advance Statements about Future Medical Treatment: A Guide for Patients.* London, Patients Association

Shears P and Stephenson G (1996) *James' Introduction to English Law* (13th edn). London, Butterworth

Singleton J and McLaren S (1995) *Ethical Foundations of Health Care.* London, CV Mosby

UKCC (1992) *Code of Professional Conduct.* London, United Kingdom Central Council for Nursing, Midwifery and Health Visiting

Weller B (1997) *Baillière's Nurses' Dictionary* (22nd edn). London, Baillière Tindall

Chapter 9 Caring for the elderly

Introduction

The operation of the NHS as we know it, is no longer as Aneurin Bevan envisaged – a service from the cradle to the grave – and the original aims of the then Labour government have become even more blurred since the introduction of the NHS and Community Care Act 1990. Among other issues, this Act has brought to the forefront the debate about whether specialised hospital care of the elderly, as opposed to the integration of care into acute medicine, would be more effective. The NHS and Community Care Act now requires the providers of care – health authorities (health boards in Scotland) – to purchase care from NHS Trusts as well as from private concerns, and sometimes requires the two groups of provider to compete for 'business' under the internal marketing process. This raises the question of whether hospitalised elderly clients would receive better care by being in a specialist department of medicine for the elderly or, as is sometimes argued, mixed-age wards in order to rationalise resources.

Related to this debate is the question of whether elderly people would receive better long-term continuing care within hospitals or in the community, that is, community care in their own homes as opposed to nursing or residential homes run by private or local authorities.

Overall health care reforms and needs, and the availability of resources, have been influenced by government policies and recommendations such as the Griffiths Report (House of Commons, Social Services Committee 1988) which was the precursor of the 1989 White Paper *Caring for People: Community Care in the next Decade and Beyond* (Department of Health 1989). These papers were, in the main, influential in the creation of policies supporting the closure of mental health hospitals and long-stay elder care institutions. Inevitably, the two documents were a major contribution to the present care of the elderly, especially of those with a mental health problem. The development of the NHS and Community Care Act 1990, together with increased patient autonomy, paved the way for the closure of long-term mental health and elder care beds in NHS institutions, care being given in preference in smaller units and private homes. Smaller units are now being seen as playing an increasing role as the main providers of care in the community for those who need full-time care.

A further underlying issue is how the *Patient's Charter* (Department of Health 1991) has affected the rights of clients and influenced decisions by health care professionals and others who direct and finance levels of patient care as well as determining the type and the quality of care that each client will receive. There is also the question of how the Charter has affected the rights of the clients, as seen by various interested parties in addition to the clients themselves. Interested parties other than the client may include pressure groups such as the Patients Association, SANE (for mental health clients) and MENCAP (for those with learning disability), along with the Parliamentary Commissioner for Administration, better known as the Ombudsman. The policy of fundholding in general practice may have an influence on how quickly a patient receives specialist treatment, the elderly often being left behind as clients with more acute illnesses are treated first. The Labour party, on winning the 1997 general election, pledged to end this anomaly of patient rights.

Background

The NHS and Community Care Act 1990 is seen by many as a turning point in the provision of care for the elderly. We are witnessing changes fuelled by the legislation that also created health care Trusts. Trusts are responsible for the direct provision of care to patients who have nursing needs. Social services departments, on the other hand, have responsibility for the provision of care to individuals who have social needs. Private concerns are also involved as providers of care for the elderly in the community by complementing health and social services; they may be funded by government sources. Care is 'purchased' from the providers by the health authorities or boards through a system known as internal marketing. The authorities or boards are expected by law to provide community health services in order to ensure the patient's continued independence in the community. Sometimes, however, problems can arise over whether a health authority/board or a local authority (the local council) should pay for clients whose health and social needs overlap.

Care of the elderly and how it is best achieved can highlight emotive issues, especially where there appears to be a deficit between clients' needs and what can be realistically provided for them. This should nevertheless be seen against a background of an increasingly healthy ageing population that is competing for limited and diminishing resources with other client groups. While it is true that the law is sometimes used by governmental agencies as a framework within which care must be provided, it is also true that there is a link between government policies and the actual level of care provided. Emphasis on care in the community has seen an argument develop over rationalisation because of the limited resources being put forward by Trusts when hospital closures and centralisation plans are implemented. Where there has been a reduction in services, recent court decisions have shown that the courts are prepared to support what they perceive as 'reasonable' measures by Trusts and social services departments. The Trusts and social services must provide the best – albeit limited – care that they can in the circumstances when available resources are taken into account. At the other end of the scale lie those who argue for the maximum institutionalised care for the elderly at whatever cost, to be provided for by the state through taxation in order to meet the original philosophy of the NHS as a cradle-to-grave provider.

It is accepted as a premise that the present-day situation is such that the financial aspect of provision of care is limited, and it is a question of deciding how far the present level can be sustained. At some point, governments, health authorities/

boards, and local authorities may have to draw the line with regard to what they can actually afford to provide. The Third Report of the House of Commons Health Committee (1996, Paras 174–96) considered community care of the elderly to be one of the government's main priorities. The recommendation was outlined as providing a single unified budget to cover the cost of social care, whether in a person's home or in a residential care or nursing home, with the opportunity for continuing care in the individual's home. This theme has been strengthened by the NHS and Community Care Act 1990 and other options for funding, including the better use of pensions and equity release schemes. The care services within the acute sector, on the other hand, appear to have been subject to previous governmental policies supporting rationalisation, centralisation and hospital closure programmes. The argument of limited resources is advanced as a justification for the resulting cuts in services.

Thinking point

> Mr Jones is 89 and receives home help. This year, the local council have put up charges for home help by 50 per cent because of budget cuts. Mr Jones cannot afford the increase but needs care and support to stay in his own home.
>
> Should he try to manage without home help? What would be the long-term effect for a frail elderly gentleman who is unable to manage?
>
> In reaching your decision, you will need to consider that, if the council reduces charges to those most in need, this may result in the home help service being cut further to balance the books, with an effect on other elderly clients.

Demographic changes – the effect on care of the elderly

The establishment of the NHS in 1946 and the improved provision of health care in the UK have become the envy of many countries. The improvement in services has resulted in people living longer than they did, while those of working age support and provide for the rising elderly population through taxation. However, economic changes over the past 30 years have taken a firm hold on British society, and many individuals who would traditionally have been carers for elderly relatives have to work for a living as a matter of necessity. The inevitable result is that the younger population are in employment and have little or no time to provide physical care for their elderly relatives. Younger families are tending to move away from their original home areas to work and live at a distance from their parents and family members. Many modern houses are designed for smaller family units and may not be suitable for elderly relatives.

The reality is that, for many reasons, a substantial number of elderly people live alone. Grundy (1989) gives a figure of 34 per cent for people aged over 65 and living on their own, and the proportion of lone households rises with age. Factfile (1996, p. 78) quotes General Household Survey figures of 50 per cent of people aged 75 and over living alone. The Royal College of Physicians report (1994) concluded that almost 50 per cent of the public expenditure budget on health and social services in any given year was spent by government on those aged 65 and above.

Thinking point

> Jessie, aged 75, needs a total hip replacement for arthritis, and elective surgery has been arranged. Jessie has had her operation cancelled because of budget cuts and short staffing.
>
> Look at the *Patient's Charter* or NHS Charter. What rights does Jessie have?

Law of negligence and elderly clients

As discussed in an earlier chapter, the law provides a framework within which appropriate care must be delivered. Government policies are in turn affected by European legislation, to which the UK acceded in 1972 by the Treaty of Rome (1957; 'The EEC Treaty'). The UK is required to implement European legislation – Directives – in their form, and there are other EC provisions that must be adapted to national law following an agreed timetable.

Care is affected by EC law in relation to the Health and Safety at Work etc. Act 1974, manual handling (the Manual Handling Operations Regulations 1992), the RIDDOR (the Reporting of Injuries, Diseases and Dangerous Occurrences Regulations 1995) and the COSHH (the Control of Substances Hazardous to Health Regulations 1994) Regulations, under which substances that may be hazardous to health are controlled.

In common law – that is, looking through cases that have gone to law and now set a precedent for the courts to go by – identified minimum standards are expected of health care professionals: the duty of care. The law expects health care professionals' as well as support staff's conduct, as measured against this yardstick, to be reasonable and to be supportable by a body of other professional carers. The effect of professional carers not meeting this standard is that they may be deemed by the courts to be in breach of this duty should they fall below expectation; if the alleged victim of a negligence goes to court, however, the onus lies on the victim to prove the negligence. The result is that the professional carer may be found liable for an act deemed to be negligent. The relevance of the law of negligence is best described as being:

essentially concerned with compensating people from the careless acts (or sometimes omissions) of others... Negligence liability will arise where the laws provide that the defendant owed the plaintiff a duty of care. (Elliot and Quinn 1996, p. 17)

Scottish law distinguishes between intentional harm *dolus* and *culpa*, which has the same meaning as negligent conduct causing property-related loss. The position in Scottish law is very similar to English law, although it places more emphasis on the need for reparation, that is, making good the harm done, making up for the harm done or compensating the victim for the harm that he or she has suffered.

This area of law, although covered mainly by tort law, or law of delict in Scotland, may also be affected by other branches of law, such as employment law. It is on this basis that one is said to be in breach of the duty of care or of employment or contractual law and that one can be sued for clinical negligence, or be in breach of the contract of employment if the carer is an employee. It is probably more difficult for the non-professional carer in the victim's home to be sued by the victim as there is normally no contract or formal agreement covering the care provided.

Elderly, frail individuals are now also protected by legislation providing for physically disabled persons, for example the Disabled Persons Act 1981 with its general provisions, and the Disability Discrimination Act 1995, which came into force in 1996, which now makes provision for better accommodation and improved access to facilities for disabled people of all ages. Other changes in legislation now affect hospitalised care to a great extent as Crown Immunity has been removed by the National Health Service (Amendment) Act 1986. Previously, under Crown Indemnity, facilities owned by the government were exempt from much of the law and could not be sued. Hospital Trusts may now be sued in the same way as any other business if their service falls short.

Furthermore, the general public are becoming increasingly aware of their rights, the law and its due process. The *Citizen's* and *Patient's Charters* have created new standards and enhanced patient rights while increasing the population's rights to previously unknown levels. The increased public awareness, supported by pressure groups and advocacy groups such as community health councils, has encouraged health care providers in both the hospital and private sectors to examine quality issues. In many cases, this has been achieved by developing policies and agreed protocols and guidelines that can be audited by both internal and external processes. The importance of efficient documentation and accurate record-keeping of practice issues cannot be underestimated in the event of future litigation.

Consent to treatment and the elderly client

The term 'treatment' is used here in its widest sense and should not be restricted only to medical treatment, but be extended to all forms of personal care as well as to medical treatment. Examples of this range of treatment include feeding, washing and rehabilitation activities that might be seen to push the elderly client beyond his or her capacity. An example of this is forcing an elderly person to walk beyond his or her capability or willingness. The general view is that all consent must be informed, that is, the client must have an explanation of the treatment and any risks involved, although this information may be justifiably restricted where medical treatment by doctors is concerned if it is in the patient's best interests. This area of law is important as an elderly client who lacks the capacity to consent or who may feel intimidated as a result of physical or mental dependency could find it difficult to refuse treatment. Despite this, the elderly have a right to informed consent, as has any other group of clients. As informed consent is a basic human right, infringement of this right can amount to abuse and find the health care worker liable to the criminal law of battery. This means that, according to the principle of informed consent, the client ordinarily has a right to be given information about the nature of treatment and any likely side-effects involved, together with the risks of the treatment. In the course of medical treatment, doctors may use clinical judgement on how much information they should disclose to clients. Doctors do have the right, supported by common law, to withhold information if, in their clinical judgement, the disclosure would be detrimental to the health of their clients.

Consent may be explicit in that clients clearly and unequivocally state their wish for the treatment or care to take place. Consent may be also implied if, by some action on their part, clients indicate that they agree. This could be a nod or an offer of a hand or a similar action to indicate co-operation: 'The ability to control any movement (lifting a finger, blinking an eye)... could be interpreted as in the affirmative, that is as a "yes"' (Ashton 1995, p. 8).

Consent is a defence to the criminal law of battery in that carers can say in their defence that they did not interfere with the client's rights because they believed that the client consented. Consent must be freely given so that the health care worker can justifiably infer that the client did give consent. It is possible to interpret that the client has freely accepted a package of care when he or she knowingly enters into an agreement to receive care or treatment.

When the elderly person is not in a position to give consent, or where consent cannot be ascertained, the law can make allowances based on the principles of beneficence and the duty of care owed to all clients. A health care professional may take the part of patient's advocate, often in collaboration with the relatives, in order to represent the client's wishes or views if they are known. As seen above, a doctor's judgement can, in some circumstances, override the patient's rights. These circumstances may include the case of 'necessity'. Necessity is where the practitioner can use the defence that, in their professional opinion and clinical judgement, where consent cannot be ascertained, the decision is taken in the best interests of the client. This is particularly relevant where matters of life and death are concerned. This principle is used when doctors have to make clinical decisions to treat a patient who is subject to a life-threatening situation and where the patient's own wishes are not known. Another example is where an incapacitated elderly person's continued presence in a particular accommodation poses a threat to themselves or other people. Then, a social worker is empowered by the National Assistance Act 1948, Section 47, to have such elderly clients removed from the unsuitable accommodation to a place of safety for their own sake or that of others. Mentally incapacitated elderly individuals are also, as are all people within the UK, subject to the Mental Health Act 1983 or the Mental Health Act (Scotland) 1984 and may be 'sectioned' by a psychiatrist and another medical officer, who frequently will be the client's own general practitioner (see Chapter 7). Registered mental nurses, approved social workers and the police also have specific powers of sectioning and removal under the provisions of the two Acts.

Social services departments normally act as advocates for incapacitated clients, but professional carers can also advocate for clients when they are not able to make a decision or where their interests are threatened. Overriding the known wishes of the patient could result in prosecution under criminal law; however, where the overriding of consent is not wilful, the law of negligence would take precedence, and the client would have to prove under the laws of tort or delict that a duty of care was breached by the defendant when the consent was overridden. The injured party – the alleged victim – could sue for damages for harm suffered.

Thinking point

Mr Roberts, aged 87, has been admitted to hospital care as he is doubly incontinent and has been neglecting himself. The other patients are complaining of the smell, and he badly needs a bath or shower but refuses when offered. How might the team approach this problem?

You will need to think about why Mr Roberts is refusing care. He may be frightened of falling in the bathroom or simply embarrassed at care being delivered by a young female nurse.

Consider how staff members may represent Mr Roberts' views to the other patients and to the doctor.

The role of the multidisciplinary team, comprising professional workers who jointly contribute to the care of the client, is important where the consent to treatment and care is blurred. Clarity of the client's wishes is often achieved by the holding of case conferences together with the client, relatives and other carers in order to arrive at decisions that are in the elder person's best interest. The purpose of multidisciplinary involvement should never be to substitute their professional interests for those of the client but to gain an agreed way to move forward with treatment or care. This is essential with the elderly since there may be multiple agencies involved in caring for the client, and it is important to ensure that their activities are co-ordinated properly in order to provide high-quality care and make best use of available resources.

Elder abuse

Elder abuse is the non-accidental injury or harm endured by an elderly dependent person; it may take many forms, be they physical, psychological or material loss. Abuse can result from a single or repeated act or acts of commission or omission on the part of a person entrusted with the care or interests of that elderly person. A useful definition is:

a single or repeated act or lack of appropriate action occurring within a relationship where there is an expectation of trust, which causes harm or distress to an older person. (Tyler 1996, p. 1)

The potential victim of elder abuse is usually subject to physical or mental incapacity and will be dependent on a relative or a professional for care. The carer is in a position of trust and therefore a position of strength in relation to the elderly client. Abuse involves lack of consent or that consent being overridden because of being obtained by deception or threats. However, while child abuse is closely monitored, with an active 'at risk' register being kept, there is no such system for recording vulnerable adults, many of them elderly, who are at risk of abuse.

The signs of abuse are not always very obvious and may be uncovered secondary to other issues, perhaps when a client is admitted to care following alleged 'falls' whose clinical findings may not be consistent with the pre-admission history and the client's health status. Where there are no obvious signs of abuse, the person who discovers or suspects abuse may be assisted by other related circumstances – which the law may interpret as circumstantial evidence – that will help in establishing whether abuse has taken place. When there are obvious signs, together with inconsistencies between the history of injury and the client's health status or immediate history of trauma, any suspected abuse should be reported immediately to a registered professional. Abuse can take place in the home or an institution, and the abuser may be a formal or informal carer or even a professional charged with the care of the client. The most common forms of abuse can be classified as follows:

- *Physical*, which is usually shown by injury of some type. This may include the criminal offence of battery, ranging from the minimum of unwanted 'touching' of the victim to the maximum of placing clients in a state of 'fear and alarm' for their immediate safety because of either an action or a threat made by the abuser. Where there is domestic violence resulting in abuse of a spouse or cohabitee, the victim may apply to the court for a non-molestation order or an injunction under either the Domestic Violence and Matrimonial Proceedings Act 1976 or the Domestic Proceedings and Magistrates Court Act 1978. Where there is actual physical harm, the matter can be reported to the police.
- *Mental or psychological*, where the effects are more difficult to show as well as more difficult to prove. Examples are bullying, ridiculing, ignoring or socially isolating the client, which could amount to false imprisonment.
- *Theft or misappropriation of property*. The abuser acquires property belonging to the client by deception or without his or her consent. This might include borrowing property with no intention to return the goods borrowed.
- *Sexual*. This can involve both physical and mental abuse. The physical aspect will involve acts of indecent assault but may stop short of full sexual intercourse, an example being unwanted intimate kissing, sexual innuendoes, dirty jokes or sexual harassment without the client's consent. Acts where full sexual intercourse takes place without the consent of the victim can amount to rape. Rape might occur when a carer forces a physically disabled partner who is incapable of consummation to have intercourse and the partner is unable to prevent it; consent is normally required for any sexual

activity even between married persons, whose consent should not be taken for granted.

Other forms of abuse may consist of the abuse of medication, malnutrition or starvation, and the provision of sub-standard treatment that is known to be harmful. This can include taking advantage of the elderly person's age and incapacity. In addition to being sued for negligence, employed carers, whether or not professional, may be in breach of their contracts of employment extra to any criminal liability.

Those who discover abuse have a duty to report it to their immediate superior if they have reasonable doubt about the alleged cause of injuries or suspect that there are other forms of abuse. The senior person, having fully investigated the issue and recorded the matter in the patient's notes, should then report the matter for further investigation and action to social workers or to the police if the client is in immediate danger from the abuser. A case conference should take place prior to discharge so that the team can ensure a care plan taking into account the victim's needs and arrange for close monitoring if the client is to return to the source of the suspected abuse.

Thinking point

> Mr Smith and his disabled wife, both 70, live together. He demands his 'marital rights to consummate' his marriage, although his wife's arthritis is such that sexual intercourse is uncomfortable and painful.
>
> On admission for rehabilitation, Mrs Smith is quite bruised and tearfully admits the situation to a member of the care team. What should now happen?

It is never easy to conclude why carers abuse victims but some reasons have been suggested: stress owing to lack of support for the carer; revenge if the carer had him- or herself been abused by the now victim; greed and the wish to acquire more property; and ignorance of the care required by a frail elderly person. The term 'abuse' can be misleading and may mask crimes such as rape, theft or assault. The reader will appreciate that, considering that a criminal offence may have taken place, any form of abuse may be managed in terms of both professional and criminal investigation, either at the same time or in sequence.

Measures for protecting property

The law provides for specific situations for dealing with management of property belonging to an elderly person who lacks the capacity, be it mental or physical, to manage his or her own affairs. Protecting the property of an elderly person may take the form of formal or less formal means depending on the need of the client.

Formal measures involve members of the legal profession. Many elderly people have a Power of Attorney drawn up, which is a formal authorisation by a person who is physically incapacitated for another suitable person to conduct their financial affairs for them. This may be for a specified length of time. An enduring Power of Attorney is similar and may be made in advance in anticipation of mental or physical incapability as it takes effect upon incapacity being present. Both types of Power must be registered with a solicitor.

The Court of Protection is another way in which the vulnerable elderly may have their interests safeguarded. An application is made to the Court on behalf of those who are not capable mentally to manage their own affairs. The Court will then appoint a 'Receiver', normally a solicitor or a professional person who usually deals with financial affairs, for example a bank manager, who will become responsible for clients' affairs. Likewise in Scotland, there is a provision for appointing a guardian along similar lines who is called a 'curator bonis', literally a 'good keeper'. The curator bonis is normally a solicitor who is a Notary Public specialising in financial, public and foreign affairs.

Less formal arrangements for managing elderly clients' affairs, particularly for those with a physical incapacity, are those of:

● Agency, in which they may temporarily nominate a family member or friend to collect their pensions for them
● Appointeeship, similar to Agency but the client making the appointment will need to put his or her wishes in writing. An example of this is when a mother nominates her son or daughter to collect money from the bank on her behalf.

There are also informal arrangements in which a dependent person can nominate a relative or friend to act as the agent to collect a pension or benefits, as long as the claimant is of sound mind. Similarly, if the recipient of the benefit becomes confused, the Benefits Agency may accept an appointee upon a written application.

Thinking point

> Have any of your clients made a Power of Attorney in order that their affairs can be managed?
>
> Do your clients have an Agent or Appointee to collect their benefits?

The elderly in acute care and the discharge process

Looking at the arguments for a speciality of acute care for the elderly, it is sometimes advanced that there is an advantage in having specialist professionals who have expertise in multiple pathology and the special problems posed by the successful discharge of an elderly client back into the community.

Within hospital care, the number of long-term beds allocated for elder care has fallen. Many Trusts are aiming at swift utilisation of the existing acute beds for general medicine, with the consequent effect of reducing the average length of stay in hospital. The role of the multidisciplinary team has become even more crucial in trying to ensure safe discharge, to comply with the requirements of the NHS and Community Care Act 1990 and to prevent 'revolving door' patients. The problems that can be caused by a delay in setting up services are highlighted by the Royal College of Physicians of London report *Ensuring Equality and Quality of Care for People* (1994, Para 313).

Conclusion: the future of care of the elderly

As people now live longer, the demand for care is increasing and problems arise if services do not match. Arguably, all the main political parties acknowledge that resources are diminishing. The considered option, according to the DoH, is that the elderly will either pay for an increased range of services or take out extra private insurance to do so. There is also a projected decrease in the number of carers (Department of Health 1996, Para 112), the corresponding forecast for an increased health care expenditure by the year 2030 being an optimistic estimate of £12.9 billion – 0.9 per cent of the country's gross domestic product. This brings into sharp focus the problem of diminishing resources and increasing number of clients who will require care in the future, a challenge for the caring professions who work with the elderly and their families.

References and further reading

Ashton G (1995) *Elderly People and the Law*. London, Age Concern/Butterworth

Bennett G and Kingston P (1995) *Elder Abuse: Concepts, Theories and Interventions*. London. Chapman & Hall

Department of Health (1989) *Caring for People: Community Care in the Next Decade and Beyond*. London, HMSO

Department of Health (1991) *The Patient's Charter*. London, HMSO

Department of Health (1996) *Third Report from the Health Committee*. London, HMSO

Elliott C and Quinn F (1996) *Tort Law*. London, Longman

Factfile (1996) *General Household Survey Figures*. London, ITC

Grundy (1989) Demographic influences on the future of family care, cited by Allen I and Perkins E (1995) *The Future of Family Care for Older People*. London, HMSO, p. 9

House of Commons (1993) *Report of the Health Committee 3rd Report: Community Care, Funding from April l993*. London, HMSO

House of Commons (1996) Report of the Health Committee. *Long-Term Care 1: Future Provision and Funding*. London, HMSO

House of Commons, Social Services Committee (1984) Griffiths NHS Management Inquiry Report. London, HMSO

Hughes B (1995) *Older People and Community Care*. Milton Keynes, Open University Press

McMahon C and Isaacs (1997) *Care of the Elderly Person: A Handbook for Care Assistants*. Oxford, Blackwell

Pritchard J (1995) *The Abuse of Older People: A Training Manual for Detection and Prevention* (2nd edn). London, Jessica Kingsley

Royal College of Nursing (1996) *Combating Abuse and Neglect of Older People: RCN Guidelines for Nurses*. London, Royal College of Nursing

Royal College of Physicians (1994) *Ensuring Quality of Care for People*. London, Royal College of Physicians

Tyler J (1996) Signs of abuse. *Nursing the Elderly*, March/April, p. 1

Chapter 10 The last word

- Introduction
- Law and ethics – their relevance to caring
- Advocacy
- Quality, audit and standards
- Consumerism and complaints
- The Ombudsman
- Role of the providers of health care and the future of the NHS
- The professions – where next?
- References and further reading

Introduction

This chapter aims to review the current state of law, morality and ethics as they relate to the care of a client by paid carers. Now that we are approaching the end of this work, there is a useful opportunity for reflection on issues that were posed in the opening chapter. Throughout the book, we have emphasised that a knowledge of the law is essential for all levels of staff who work within the broad sector of health care provision. Whether a carer is involved in looking after someone as a paid professional, a support worker or a family member or close friend, there is a need to act in the client's best interests. Health care professionals are frequently called upon to act as advocates to ensure clients' well-being and to represent their expressed interests. Professional codes and rules should reflect the need for professionals and lay carers to respect the individual patient's interests, although these may be modified or limited by other competing interests or limitation of resources.

Publication of the Labour government's plans concerning the NHS, in the form of two White Papers covering England and Scotland, places an emphasis on the delivery of quality care that can be audited. An increased understanding of clients' rights and a rising movement towards consumerism on the part of the

161

public as a whole appear to have resulted in an increased number of complaints within the NHS. For clients, or their representatives, who fail to reach agreement on the handling of complaints, an approach may be made to the Parliamentary Commissioner for Administration, Health Service, better known as the Ombudsman.

As consumerism extends further, and public expectations of the care and treatment that can be delivered increase, the care that can be achieved within the NHS is assessed. As the NHS evolves and changes, the health care professions themselves also have to adjust their stance on some issues; this is considered briefly at the end of the chapter.

Law and ethics – their relevance to caring

The question arises of what is the relevance to care of the law and moral rules, often expressed as ethics. It is clear that the law, acting as a broad reflection of the moral values held by society in the UK, provides a framework within which care is provided: 'As far as the law is concerned there must clearly be a close connection with morality since they have concepts in common such as justice, rights, rules, responsibility, and many others' (Downie and Calman 1994, p. 41). Ethical behaviour on the part of registered health care professionals is the outcome of the moral behaviour expected to be displayed in the course of professionals' duties. Both the law and formal codes of ethics allow redress to those who feel aggrieved with action being taken by society in the case of the law – or the professional bodies if a code of conduct is breached by the practitioner. The regulatory effect of the law is seen when the professional carer or support worker is in breach of the rules. They may find that they are liable to be prosecuted under criminal law, sued under civil law (tort/delict) or have action taken against them under industrial relations law and procedure.

However, all those employed to deliver care are faced with ethical decision-making on a small scale in the course of their duties. Singer defines a practical ethic as 'relevant if it is one that any thinking person must face' (1993, p. vii). All health care workers, whether they are registered professionals, students or support workers, need to be thinking carers. Here, the law and codes provide guidance, and the supervision of unqualified staff by a professional should result in care informed by ethical and legal considerations.

An ethical question still remains that affects both the individual health care worker and society as a whole. The ethical principle of justice is the one linked to resource allocation and health care rationing. Should life-saving treatment be provided for one patient or client alone when available resources could benefit a much wider clientele? Public debate over 'Child B' in the mid-1990s bought this matter into sharp focus: should scarce resources be used to treat a child who was suffering from almost certainly terminal leukaemia or be used to treat others with a similar condition whose disease was not so advanced? The question was widely debated, but only one side could be heard at the time, as the health care Trust involved were bound by client confidentiality. Despite the one-sided nature of the debate at the time, matters such as this very sad case are now a matter for public scrutiny.

Advocacy

Advocacy is the representation of a client's wishes by a health care worker to a third party and is closely related to the concept of empowerment. Despite this, clients should, whenever possible, represent themselves supported by health care workers who are empowering the clients to make their own decisions: 'Empowerment means helping the less competitive to compete more effectively' (Gomm 1993, p. 136). In some areas, the whole of health care delivery may be directed towards this one aim – enabling clients to act for themselves at one level or another. For those clients who are profoundly mentally or physically disabled, this may not be possible, although the law only condones compulsory treatment under some sections of the Mental Health Act 1983 and the Mental Health Act (Scotland) 1984. For this group of clients, health care professionals play an important part in representing clients' best interests and helping clients to understand their treatment and care. For a client who is mentally disordered and involved in criminal proceedings, the health care worker may act as the client's advocate by taking 'appropriate adult' status under the Police and Criminal Evidence Act 1984 (see Chapter 7).

As discussed in several chapters in this book, issues of informed consent can prove problematic, and each case will differ, the principle of mental competency being the deciding factor. Government policy on health care stresses the importance of clients taking part in health care decisions affecting them. In all forms of advocacy, clients' wishes must remain paramount, health care workers acting as a support to the clients.

Quality, audit and standards

The White Paper *The New NHS: Modern, Dependable* (Department of Health 1997), together with its Scottish counterpart *Designed to Care: Renewing the National Health Service in Scotland* (Scottish Office 1997), place great importance on the future quality of care delivery within the NHS. Many Trusts, in both the acute and community sectors, have developed standards of care that can be audited to give an overall picture of the success of care delivery – or its failure. If, on audit, standards of care are not being met, the managers of care can then take steps to remedy the problem. Although these measures are not enshrined in law, they fall within the context of professional practice and accountability:

Professional and statutory bodies have a vital role in setting and promoting standards, but shifting the focus towards quality will also require practitioners to accept responsibility for developing and maintaining standards within their local NHS organisations. (Department of Health 1997, p. 47)

While the development of standards and quality care on an auditable basis is comparatively easy within the NHS, what of the private sector? This sector is taking a greater role in the provision of long-term health care, a situation likely to continue in the future. Homes registered under the Registered Homes Act 1984 are liable to regular inspection by the local authority, and registration can be withdrawn if the home fails to meet the provisions of the Act. The Act does lay out some standards, but they are in the main very basic, reflecting the fundamental needs of a dependent client rather than quality of care. Many residential and nursing homes are run to a very high standard, but, in an increasingly competitive market, some cut corners, with a consequent loss of quality and to the potential detriment of both residents and staff. Redress for aggrieved clients or their relatives may require recourse to legal action against the home via either the civil or even the criminal route.

Consumerism and complaints

Since the 1970s and the European Community Act of 1972, which legalised British membership of the EC, there has been a growth of what is generally called consumerism in many aspects of life. In health care, this means that patients or clients are now more prepared to complain or go to litigation – law – for redress where they would previously have taken no action. There has also been a growth in consumer law now developing as a speciality within legal practice. For example, statutes such as the Consumer Protection Act 1974, the Fair Trading Act 1975 and the Sale of Goods Act 1979 have protected the interests of the ordinary person in the street. The Legal Aid Act 1979 made it easier for poorer people to sue, although legal aid is now being restricted in some areas of law. The EC addressed the specific area of strict liability covering injury arising from defective goods, including medicinal products, by introducing the EC Directive of 1985 on Product Liability.

These changes shifted the focus from an overall picture to a more individual one, and the introduction of the *Citizen's Charter* and the *Patient's Charter* (the *Patient's Charter* is soon to be replaced by an NHS Charter) stated the expectations that individual consumers of health care could anticipate. Stephen Dorrell, then Health Minister, stated that:

Furthermore, when they [NHS providers] have made their decisions, they must also expect to explain them to a public in language which the public understands. The language of public service must not be impenetrable jargon of the expert – it must be the language of the servant giving account of himself to his master. (Dorrell quoted by Williams 1996, p. 20)

More emphasis on consumer rights, allied to a greater degree of openness, has led to a rising number of complaints being made about NHS treatment and care. The link between increased consumerism and the rise in complaints is considered by Wilder (1997, p. 28).

Within the NHS, complaints can be a useful way of improving quality and are seen as the clients' way of expressing their opinion of how the service is being delivered. Complaints should not be regarded as a nuisance but as a source of information on what can go wrong and how the service can be improved. As complaints can have a negative effect on morale, clients should be encouraged also to make positive comments in order to acknowledge effective service provision. If a client wishes to make a complaint about treatment or care, whether in hospitals or the community, they or their relatives can take advantage of leaflets describing the procedure that have been developed by NHS providers.

Under the new NHS complaints procedure and the Hospital Complaints Procedure Act 1985, complaints should normally be made by patients or their representatives (with the client's permission) within 6 months, although this time limit can be waived if the reason for the delay is acceptable. Informal complaints are normally made by clients at the point of delivery, and the health professional who receives the complaint will address the problem promptly or refer the problem to the departmental manager for immediate address. If complainants are not satisfied, they have the right to complain further, in writing. At this stage, the complaint is known as a formal complaint. Formal complaints are normally dealt with by a complaints manager who is usually the Chief Executive or a designated manager within the organisation. The complaints manager has to consider the following issues when making an investigation: whether the complaint is a disciplinary issue; whether it is professional misconduct, in which case it may be reported to the responsible regulating body; whether it requires an independent inquiry if it is a particularly serious incident; whether there should be an organisational review of practice as a whole; and, last, whether the incident should be reported to the police.

In the community, community health Trusts have structures similar to those of acute (hospital) Trusts, while the complaints about general practitioners and their staff should be directed through the family health practitioner committee.

If a complaint cannot be resolved, it may be adequate for it to be dealt with at local level by an independent review panel. The panel can only recommend action; it has no legal power to enforce its decision.

The Ombudsman

A small number of complaints end up with the Ombudsman. The Ombudsman may investigate complaints against the NHS from members of the public regarding their dissatisfaction with the way in which they have been treated. The Ombudsman is independent, and the service is free. Complaints should be made within a year of the date the complainant became aware of events. The local complaints procedure must be followed and exhausted before it can reach the Ombudsman, who can investigate complaints related to:

a. a poor service;
b. failure to purchase or provide a service you are entitled to receive;
c. maladministration – that is administrative failure such as:
    - avoidable delays
    - not following proper procedures
    - rudeness or discourtesy
    - not explaining decisions
    - not answering your complaint fully or promptly
d. complaints about the care and treatment provided by a doctor, nurse or other trained professional
e. other complaints about family doctors (GPs), or about dentists, pharmacists or opticians providing a NHS service locally. (Health Service Commissioner 1997)

Any other issues outside this remit may be referred to the court or industrial tribunal.

During the Ombudsman's investigation of the complaint, all papers and documents relating to the case are likely to be inspected, and staff can be summoned to give evidence. All matters in the complaint are then considered, and recommendations are made. Copies of the Ombudsman's report are then sent to the local MP and the complainant, and a summary is forwarded to the Trust against whom the complaint has been made. A summary is also sent to the press, so publicity is likely to feature in the investigation.

Health care consumers who go to court to sue for negligence must prove that they suffered on three accounts: that they were owed a duty of care, that there was a breach of that duty, and that they suffered harm as a result.

Role of the providers of health care and the future of the NHS

The NHS is at the core of health care provision in the UK. Increasingly, however, private concerns contribute directly and indirectly through the tendering process, for example in the provision of agency staff.

Since the inception of the NHS, now more than 50 years ago, we have seen it transformed from the ideology of a 'cradle-to-grave' health care provision to being the main provider of care in essential, acute services. Because of limited resources and an increasing demand for health care free at the point of delivery, it has not always been possible, for economic reasons, to see Bevan's vision through. In fact, governments of different political stances have regularly restructured the NHS, with varying degrees of success. Because of increasing costs in the running and delivery of health care, government policy has encouraged private sector involvement. The announcement, in 1998, of the use of the private finance initiative (PFI) to build new hospitals is an example. Using the PFI, the private sector will build new hospitals and then lease them back to the NHS for a period of 25 years. What has not been made clear is what will happen at the end of the 25-year period – will private companies reclaim the hospitals to run them themselves on a fee-paying basis?

One of the most fundamental changes affecting the role of the NHS springs from the NHS and Community Care Act 1990 and its related legislation. This has committed health care provision generally to a far more community-based model of care than has previously been the case. As we have seen, the care of the mentally handicapped only entered the NHS as a quirk of history; elderly people in the days before the NHS were largely cared for in the community. For the elderly, prior to the NHS and the provision of long-stay care, the humiliation of the workhouse infirmary resulted in the majority being cared for at home until their death. In the modern UK, the idea of full-time care at home is no longer a general possibility as more women – who give most of the care – are employed on either a full- or a part-time basis. Thus much of the care of the frail elderly has moved into the private sector, with an expanding sector of care provision. Physically disabled individuals are no longer catered for within the NHS provision of long-stay beds; in their case, care has been developed by social services, voluntary agencies and the development of small group homes within the community.

As the NHS has become more and more business orientated, managers have adopted practices more closely allied to industry than the former pattern of health care delivery. Audit has provided a wealth of information on efficiency, and it is now possible to judge one hospital's performance against another's in selected procedures. The difficulty is that this approach relies entirely on known demand, the well-known 'waiting list' figures. The services with a less predictable demand cannot be quantified in the same way, although some direction can be given by the analysis of statistics relating to seasonal demands – for example in chest medicine – allowing a degree of planning to take place.

The incoming government, led by Tony Blair, published its intentions in late 1997 towards the NHS in the form of two White Papers – *The New NHS: Modern, Dependable* (Department of Health 1997) for England and *Designed to Care; Renewing the National Health Service in Scotland* (Scottish Office 1997) for Scotland. The move towards community care given in the previous (Conservative) government's NHS and Community Care Act 1990 is reinforced and strengthened by the planned development of primary care groups, which will eventually become primary health care Trusts. These Trusts are envisaged as being formed by general practitioners and health care professionals – nurses being particularly mentioned – working together within the community. The use of technology is also promoted to speed the flow of information from the hospital to the general practitioner and vice versa. A close working relationship with the local authorities is seen as the key to quality care provision. As has been discussed throughout this book, much of social and personal care already lies within the remit of local authorities, often on a statutory basis, with close collaboration between health and social services now being an essential feature.

The health care system within Northern Ireland, where health and social services have been united for many years, may possibly alter in the future following the repeal of the 1920 Ireland Act and the separate legislation currently in force within Northern Ireland.

The professions – where next?

In this scenario of change, it is inevitable that the health care professions and those registered as professionals will have to adjust and change in the light of planned changes for the NHS itself. Nursing forms the largest profession within health care and is at the forefront of the projected changes. In recent years, nurse education has entered the university framework, joining the other health care professions. This change has been controversial but has in reality only been the first move in putting nursing on an equal footing with other health care professions in the workplace. At present, nurses may register after studying for a diploma level qualification at a university; many choose to build on this qualification and gain a degree in either nursing or an allied subject. In order to achieve the same qualification at registration as the majority of the members of the multidisciplinary team, it is probable that nursing degrees will become the basic qualification in the future. Many registered nurses holding the former 'ward sister' grade are now managers of care within the acute sector, co-ordinating care delivery by members of the multidisciplinary team. The divisions between nursing and the work of junior doctors is becoming more blurred:

A quiet revolution is occurring in the division of labour between the professions of medicine and nursing, created partly by the requirements to reduce junior doctor's work… Nurses in particular are taking on clinical work that has traditionally been done by doctors. (Dowling *et al.* 1996, p. 1211)

In all professions allied to medicine – including nursing – evidence-based practice is becoming the norm rather than the exception. The professions are developing standards and guidelines for practice grounded in research and supported by a thriving publications industry, and these can be used to argue the case when professional disputes arise. The old argument that nurses, among the other professions, were cheaper than doctors is no longer valid when more senior grades are examined.

In recognition of this advancement in knowledge on the part of the professions allied to medicine, the NHS (Primary Care) Act 1997 allows health care professionals to join the tendering process for the provision of services. At present, this is limited to pilot schemes, but it could expand in the future.

All these developments bring forward the notion of autonomous practice by a registered professional.

At present, professional practice is covered by vicarious liability, in that the employer covers claims against professional practice provided that the employee was acting within his or her role. Reference to the job description will often help clarification of exactly what is expected of the professional. As practice becomes more autonomous, whether within the community or within the acute services, it is likely that responsibility for the insurance of practice will have to be taken, at least partially, by the individual practitioner. This reflects the pattern of doctors and independent therapists, who indemnify their practice. Certainly, as the number of support workers is likely to rise, the registered professional will take on more and more of a supervisory and managerial role in order to deliver high-quality care to the client, becoming responsible for the actions of those who are being supervised.

References and further reading

Brazier M (1992) *Medicines, Patients and the Law*. London, Penguin

Brown P and Sparks R (1990) *Beyond Thatcherism: Social Policy, Politics and Society*. Milton Keynes, Open University Press

Department of Health (1997) *The New NHS: Modern, Dependable*. London, HMSO

Dowling S, Martin R, Skidmore P, Doyal L, Cameron A and Lloyd S (1996) Nurses taking on junior doctor's work: a confusion of accountability. *British Medical Journal* **312**: 1211–14

Downie R and Calman K (1994) *Healthy Respect: Ethics in Health Care* (2nd edn). Oxford, Oxford University Press

Dyer C (ed.) (1993) *Doctors, Patients and the Law*. Oxford, Blackwell Scientific

Gomm R (1993) Issues of power. In Walmsley J, Reynolds J, Shakespeare P and Woolfe R (eds) *Health, Welfare and Practice: Reflecting on Roles and Relationships*. Milton Keynes, Open University Press/Sage

Health Service Commissioner (1997) *What can the Ombudsman Investigate?* www.health.ombudsman.org.uk/hsc/what

Lowe R and Woodroffe G (1991) *Consumer Law and Practice* (3rd edn). London, Sweet & Maxwell

McHale J, Fox M and Murphy J (1997) *Health Care Law: Text and Materials*. London, Sweet & Maxwell

McHale J, Tingle J and Peysner J (1998) *Law and Nursing*. Oxford, Butterworth Heinemann

Mohan J (1995) *A National Health Service: The Restructuring of Health Care in Britain Since 1979.* Basingstoke, Macmillan

Pollitt C (1996) *Managerialism and the Public Services – Cuts or Cultural Change in the 1990s.* Oxford, Blackwell Business

Pullen F (1995) Advocacy: a specialist practitioner role. *British Journal of Nursing* 4(5): 275–8

Ranade W (1994) *A Future for the NHS: Health Care in the 1990s.* London, Longman

Scottish Office (1997) *Designed to Care: Renewing the National Health Service in Scotland.* Edinburgh, Stationery Office

Singer P (1993) *Practical Ethics* (2nd edn). Cambridge, Cambridge University Press

Wilder G (1997) Pay back time *Health Service Journal*, **107**(5545): 28–31

Williams K (1996) *A Practical Approach to Caring.* Edinburgh, Longman

Appendix Useful addresses

Statutory bodies

Commission for Racial Equality

England:
Elliot House,
10-12 Allington Street,
London SW1E 5EH

Scotland:
100 Princes Street,
Edinburgh,
EH2 3AA

Community Health Councils
See your local telephone directory

Health and Safety Executive
Information Centre,
Broad Lane,
Sheffield S3 7HQ
*(or see your local telephone directory for
local offices)*

Professional bodies

British Association of Occupational
Therapists Ltd
6–8 Marshalsea Road,
London SE1 1HL

Chartered Society of Physiotherapy
14 Bedford Row,
London WC1R 4ED

Royal Pharmaceutical Society
1 Lambeth High Street,
London SE1 7JN

United Kingdom Central Council for
Nursing, Midwifery and Health
Visiting (UKCC)
23 Portland Place,
London W1N 4JT

Trade unions/professional support

Royal College of Nursing of the United
Kingdom (RCN)
20 Cavendish Square,
London W1M OAB

UNISON
1 Mabledon Place,
London WC1H 9AJ

Charitable/non-profit-making bodies
*(You are requested to include a stamped
addressed envelope with any enquiry that
you make)*

Age Concern
Astral House,
1268 London Road,
London SW16 4ER

Carers National Association
20 Glasshouse Yard,
London EC1A 4JS

Childline
2nd Floor,
Royal Mail Building,
Studd Street,
London N1 OQW

Disabled Living Foundation
380–384 Harrow Road,
London W9 2HU

Mental After Care Association (MACA)
25 Bedford Row,
London WC1B 3HW

The Mental Health Charity (SANE)
2nd Floor,
199–205 Old Marylebone Road,
London NW1 5QP

National Society for the Prevention of
Cruelty to Children
National Centre,
42 Curtain Road,
London EC2A 3NH

Patients Association
18 Victoria Park Square,
London E2 9PF

Royal Scottish Society for the
Prevention of Cruelty to Children
(RSPCC)
Melville House,
41 Polwarth Terrace
Edinburgh EH11 1NU

RSPCC
Annfield Family Resource Centre,
15 Annfield Place,
Dennistoun,
Glasgow G31 1XE

Royal Society for Mentally
Handicapped Children and Adults
(MENCAP)
Mencap National Centre,
123 Golden Lane,
London EC1Y ORT

Scottish Association for Mental Health
38 Gardners Crescent,
Edinburgh EH3 8DQ

Scottish Downs Syndrome Association,
158–160 Balgreen Road,
Edinburgh EH11 3AU

Index

Undergraduate Lending Library WITHDRAWN